Kitchen Clinic

Home Remedies for Common Ailments

Dr. Shiv Charan Sharma
Dr. Syed Aziz Ahmad

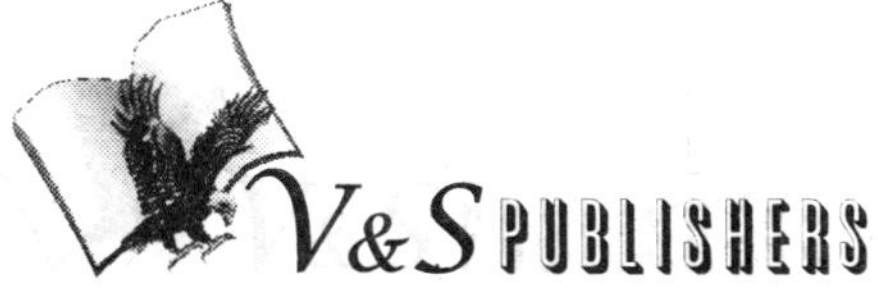

Published by:

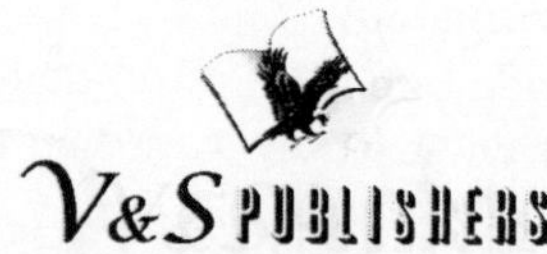

F-2/16, Ansari Road, Daryaganj, New Delhi-110002
☎ 011-23240026, 011-23240027 • *Fax:* 011-23240028
Email: info@vspublishers.com • *Website:* www.vspublishers.com

Regional Office : Hyderabad
5-1-707/1, Brij Bhawan (Beside Central Bank of India Lane)
Bank Street, Koti, Hyderabad - 500 095
☎ 040-24737290
E-mail: vspublishershyd@gmail.com

Branch Office : Mumbai
Jaywant Industrial Estate, 1st Floor–108, Tardeo Road
Opposite Sobo Central Mall, Mumbai – 400 034
☎ 022-23510736
E-mail: vspublishersmum@gmail.com

Follow us on: 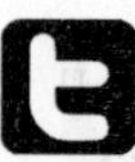  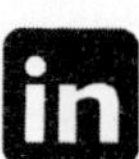

All books available at **www.vspublishers.com**

ISBN 978-93-81384-5-8-9
Edition: 2019

Printed at : Param Offseters Okhla New Delhi-110020

Dedication

In loving memory of my late father who dedicated his life for the cause of Ayurveda & inspired me to know medicinal plants.

—Dr. S.C. Sharma

Acknowledgement

We express our deep sense of gratitude to old men, *bhagats, hakims, vaidyas,* and other villagers, without whose cooperation, this work would not have been possible. We are thankful to Dr. Rakesh ravi and Dr. A.M. Tripathi for valuable suggestions, and Mr. R.C. Sharma for quick typing of the manuscript.

—Dr. S. C. Sharma
—Dr. S. A. Ahmad

INTRODUCTION

Kitchen is a functional as well as a storage place in a house where raw materials are used to prepare food, domestic dishes, non-alcoholic beverages etc. Most of raw material are plants and their products, such as chilli, coriander, cumin, dill, fennel, turmeric, cloves, wheat flour, vegetables, onion etc. Majority of them have therapeutic value and provide fairly reliable remedies that are safe and less expensive. They can be used in odd hours of night and in emergency to cure coughs, cuts, sore throats, various types of pains, earache, toothache etc. as alternative medicines.

Today, pollution has played havoc with our lives, causing innumerable diseases, mental tension and stress. Therefore, nature's cure or herbal medicines are quite fruitful and beneficial to human health. Recently, there has been a great liking for anything herbal, as it is deemed pure, fresh and without any side effects. Unfortunately, we are gradually forgetting the use of these indigenous herbs and medicines, as they are not commonly used by us. The information contained in this book is author's interesting, fruitful and based on our traditional knowledge and extensive experience down the centuries.

It is hoped that our readers will cure the ailments of the members of their family, neighbours and friends with the prescriptions contained in this book.

The information available in this book has been collected from experienced people, *sadhus, hakims, vaidyas* and others, who worked as folk-healers in the past.

Contents

1

SALAD PLANTS

1. Carrot (Gajar)

Botanical name : *Daucus carota* L.
Family : (Apiaceae Umbelliferae)
Sanskrit name : Gunjan
Plant part used : Root

Identification

An erect, biennial herb with fleshy conical tap root. Leaves decompound. Infloresce in termind compound umbel, white. Fruits cremocarp with hooked spines.

Distribution

It is a native of Mediterranean region from where it spread throughout the world. It is cultivated in Europe, Asia and Africa. In India, it is grown in majority of the states.

Chemical Composition

On an average, the fresh root contains 86% moisture, 0.9% proteins and 0.1% mineral matter. It also contains carotene, (a precursor of Vitamin A) and appreciable amounts of thiamine and riboflavin.

Medicinal Uses

1. ***To cure eye trouble***—Take the juice of fresh root in a cup. Mix it with 250 gm of fennel and 10 gm of sugar. Take this mixture with milk at night before sleep.

2. ***To heal wounds or sores***—Boil the roots and prepare a poultice. Place it over the wounds or sores and tie it with white thin piece of muslin cloth. Repeat it for at least 3-5 days.

3. ***To make heart strong***—Boil fresh roots and prepare paste. Place the paste open under the moonlight. After adding few drops of rose water and sufficient sugar, take it early in the morning.

4. ***To cure headache***—Boil the fresh roots and extract the juice. Place 2 or 3 drops of juice in the nostril. Repeat 2 times after an interval of 15 minutes.

5. ***To remove intestinal diseases***—A diet supplemented by raw carrots each day helps cleaning up constipation, promoting some looseness of the stool, providing relief in piles and sprue and killing worms in the intestine.

6. ***To have a check on Cancer***—Carrot, a well-known source of anti-cancer nutrient, ß-carotene. It helps keep off cancer if consumed regularly.

7. ***To remove kidney stones***—Make a cavity in the root and fill it with the seeds of turnip and radish. Close the cavity and then boil it. Take it twice a day. Stones will get dissolved.

8. ***To heal the burns***—Pour ice water first on the burnt part of the body. Dip thin cloth in carrot juice and tie lightly over the burnt part. Repeat it for 3 days.

9. ***To cure dysentery***—Boil the roots and extract juice. Take one cup juice thrice a day.

10. ***To improve eye sight***—It is a potent source of vitamin A, which is a boon for eyes. One should eat 3/4 carrots daily.

11. ***Vitamin E***—Carrots' leaves are a great source of vitamin E. Its juice is prepared & taken as per need.

12. ***To maintain Osmoregulation***—It is such in alkaline elements, which purify and revitalise the blood and it tone up the whole system & helps maintain acid/base balance of the body.

2. Cucumber (Kheera)

Botanical name : *Cucumis sativus* L.

Family : Cucurbitaceae

Sanskrit name : Sukasa

Plant part used : Fruit

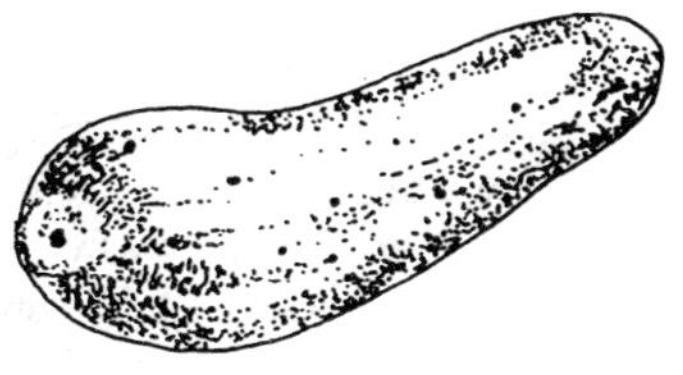

Identification

Annual prostrate herb. Leaves broadly cordate-ovate, villose-hispid. Fruits oblong, yellowish-green, glabrous.

Distribution

It is a native of northern India. It was cultivated in Egypt, Greece and China in ancient time. Now it is cultivated throughout the world.

Chemical Composition

On an average, the fruit contains 93% moisture, 2.5% carbohydrates, 0.1% fat, 0.7% minerals, 0.2% proteins and 0.6% fibres. It is also a source of potassium, calcium and vitamin B and C.

Medicinal Uses

1. ***To relieve tired and inflamed eyes***—Fruit is crushed to make poultice. It is applied in fine cloth on the lids for half an hour.
2. ***To cure insect sting***—Thin slices of the fruit are made. They are placed over the place of sting one after another. They will draw sting poison.
3. ***To dissolve kidney stones***—Take raw cucumber as salad daily with meal. It will help dissolve the stones in kidney.
4. ***To check assimilation of uric acid***—Uric acid causes stone formation, rheumatic problems etc. Taking kheera daily enhances urine production, thus washing away uric acid from the body.

3. Lemon (Neebu)

Botanical name : *Citrus limon* (L.) Burm.f.
Family : Rutaceae
Sanskrit name : Maha nimbu
Plant part used : Fruit

Identification

A small thorny tree. Leaves ovate, petioles winged. Flowers tinged red. Fruit ovoid, yellow, rind thin.

Distribution

Lemon is a native of south-eastern Asia, most probably north-western India. It reached Europe through Arabs in the 10th century. Now it is cultivated throughout the world.

Chemical Composition

Fruit consists of 87.4% moisture, 0.9% proteins, 10.6% carbohydrates and 0.4% minerals. It also has organic acids (citric acid, malic acid), essential oils, glycosides, anthocyanins, ß-carotene and vitamin C.

Medicinal Uses

1. ***To check bleeding***—For profuse bleeding occuring from any part of the body, place a few drops of lemon juice there. Bleeding will definitely be stopped.
2. ***To reduce obesity***—Take juice in a glass of water each day after dinner.
3. ***To cure sore-throat***—Place lemon juice in a little warm water. Gargle several times each day.
4. ***To relieve upset stomach***—Cut lemon peals into small pieces and dry them. Place some of them in 2 cups of water and boil for 30 minutes. Drink twice a day.
5. ***To remove eczema***—First rub it at the site of eczema and then place the lemon juice there. Repeat it for 2 or 3 times a day.

6. ***To prepare a face wash***—Take lemon juice, add sugar and borax in equal amounts. Mix them to make a paste. Rub it on the face to remove pimples and black spots.

7. ***To strengthen resistance***—Juice of lemon gives good amount of vitamin C, which helps in fighting disease, cures cold & cough, gives luster to skin and strength to gums.

8. ***To get relief in piles***—Cut fruit into two equal halves and place 5 gm katha (Acacia catechu) powder on each half. Keep them open at whole right. Suck the juice of both halves in the morning for a week.

4. Onion (Pyaz)

Botanical name : *Allium cepa* L.
Family : Liliaceae
Sanskrit name : Palandu
Plant part used : Bulb (underground stem)

Identification

Biennial crop with large bulb. Root system is shallow and fibrous. Leaves radical, hollow, bifarius. Flowers many, white, in dense umbels. Fruit its capsules sub-globose.

Distribution

Native to south-west Asia and eastern Mediterranean region. Now cultivated in all parts of the world. In India, chiefly grown in Maharashtra, Tamil Nadu, Andhra Pradesh, Bihar and Punjab.

Chemical Composition

On an average, a mature onion contains 87% moisture, 11% carbohydrates, 1.2% proteins, 0.4% minerals, 0.6% fibres and also has traces of thiamine, nicotinic acid, riboflavin and vitamin C. The pungency of onion is due to a volatile oil, allyl propyl disulphide.

Medicinal Uses

1. ***To cure night blindness***—Two drops of onion juice is placed in the eyes in early morning and at night before sleep.
2. ***To remove kidney stones***—Take onion as salad with meal. The stones in kidney or in urinary bladder break and pass with urine.
3. ***To relieve earache***—Take juice of the bulb, warm it and put 2 or 3 drops in the ear. The ache will go soon.
4. ***To cure nasal bleeding***—Put three or four drops of onion juice in the nostrils. Repeat it thrice a day.

5. ***To treat piles***—Prepare juice of the bulb. Mix the juice with sugar in equal amounts. Take the mixture thrice a day at an interval of 4 hours.

6. ***To remove pimples***—Take 10 gm juice of white onion, honey 5 gm and salt 1 gm. Mix them and then rub it on the face.

7. ***To cure cholera***—Mix onion juice and mint juice (Mentha longifolia) in equal amounts. Warm the mixture. Take it regularly after an interval of half an hour.

8. ***To kill lice in hair***—Prepare juice of the bulb. Apply it over the head. Lices will be killed.

9. ***To reduce hypertension***—Take onion as salad daily with the meal. It helps control the high blood pressure.

10. ***To destroy worms in intestine***—Take onion as salad with the meal. It destroys the intestinal parasites.

11. ***To lower the blood sugar***—Take onion as salad. It is helpful for lowering the sugar level in diabetic patients.

12. ***To cure insect stings***—Apply juice of the bulb over the site of insect sting or bite. Leave it for 3 hours.

13. ***To treat snake bite***—Mix 3 spoonfuls of onion juice and the same amount of mustard oil. Consume it regularly at an interval of half an hour.

14. ***To treat urinary problems***—For burning sensation in urine, 6 gms of onion should be boiled in half litre. It is then cooled and given to patients. Onion rubbed in water and mixed with sugar is useful in urine retention.

15. ***An Aphrodisiac***—It increases libido and strengthens the reproductory organs and 2 table spoons of white onion juice, 2 table spoons honey and one table spoon adrak juice mixed together and taken 3 times a day.

5. Radish (Mooli)

Botanical name : *Raphanus sativus* L.
Family : Brassiaceae Cruciferae
Sanskrit name : Mulaka
Plant part used : Root and green leaves

Identification

A quick-growing annual or biennial bristly herb with fleshy root. Leaves lyratepinnate or pinnatifid. Flowers white or lilac. The fruit is a fleshy siliqua with a long conical beak.

Distribution

The radish, native to western Asia, was cultivated in Egypt, Greece and Rome. Japan and China are the major producer. It is cultivated all over India.

Chemical Composition

On an average radish consists of 94.4% moisture, 3.4% carbohydrates, 0.7% protein, 0.1% fat, 0.6% minerals and 0.8% fibres. It also contains the trace of vitamin A, thiamine, riboflavin, nicotinic acid and vitamin C. The characteristic pungent flavour of radish is due to the presence of volatile isothiocyanates.

Medicinal Uses

1. ***To reduce trouble in urination***—Take radish as a salad with daily meal. It will help to reduce trouble in urination.
2. ***To cure jaundice***—Prepare juice of the green leaves and mix some sugar. Filter it. Take the filtrate 2 times a day for a week.
3. ***To treat piles***—Make the green leaves dry under shade and then crush them to powder. Mix equal amount of sugar. Take the mixture once a day. After one month piles will go.

4. ***To provide scorpion sting remedy***—Place juice of the root over the site of scorpion sting. It will provide relief immediately.

5. ***To give relief in earache***—Mix Juice of the leaves and sesame oil in equal amount. Boil the mixture till only the oil is left in the pan. Cool it, then filter and store it in a bottle. Whenever there is pain in the ear, put 2 or 3 drops after mild warming. The pain will disappear immediately.

6. ***To cure spleen trouble***—Cut root lengthwise and place Ammonium chloride over it. Keep it open for a night and then take it early in the morning. Repeat it for a month.

7. ***To digest starchy foods***—Take the raw radish as salad with the meal for easier digestion of starches.

8. ***To stop hiccup***—Boil some part of the root in water. Filter it. Take it to stop hiccup.

9. ***To check leucoderma***—A paste of seeds in vinegar is applied on the white spots continuously for a month.

10. ***To check chest trouble***—A syrup prepared by mixing a teaspoonful of fresh radish juice and equal quantity of honey plus a pinch of black salt 3 times daily is useful in bronchial disorder of whooping cough.

6. Sugar Beet (Chukandar)

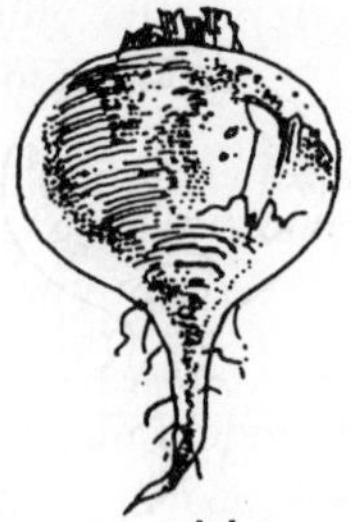

Botanical name : *Beta vulgaris* L.

Family : Chenopodiaceae

Sanskrit name : Palanki

Plant part used : Roots

Identification

A glabrous herb with fleshy root. Leaves ovate to oblong-ovate. Flowers green, many, in open ponicles.

Distribution

It is a native of northern Europe. It is now cultivated throughout the world. In India it is commonly grown in North India, Maharashtra and South India.

Chemical Composition

On an average, the root contains 83.8% moisture, 1.7% protein, 13.6% carbohydrates, 0.1% fat and 0.8% mineral matter. There are also traces of calcium, potassium, iron and vitamin B_1 and C.

Medicinal Uses

1. ***To give relief in cancer***—Take fresh root as salad. It gives relief in cancer due to a tumour inhibiting gradient present in it.
2. ***To treat anaemia***—Take raw beet roots daily. It will increase the number of red blood corpuscles in an anaemic patient.
3. ***As a source of Iron***—Prepare juice of the roots. Take a glass of juice daily. It has high content of iron, which reactivates R.B.C. and supplies fresh oxygen to the body.
4. ***To check piles***—Eating beetroot is also useful for constipation and piles. If used daily, it prevents habitual constipation, thus helping in piles.
5. ***To clean kidney & gall bladder***—It has properties to make kidney & gall bladder clean.

7. Tomato (Tamatar)

Botanical name : *Lycopersicon esculentum Mill.*
Family : Solanaceae
Sanskrit name : Tamatar
Plant part used : Fruit

Identification

A weak-stemmed, trailing, many-branched, short-lived perennial herb.

Distribution

A native of Peru and Ecuador, it spread to Mexico and Europe. It was introduced to south-east Asian countries. It grows throughout warm temperate and tropical regions.

Chemical Composition

On average, tomato consists of 93% moisture, 3.6% carbohydrates, 1.9% protein, 0.1 fat, 0.6% minerals, 0.7% fibre. Vitamins A, B_1, B_2 and C are also present. A rich source of potassium.

Medicinal Uses

1. ***To control high blood pressure***—Take tomato as salad with daily meal. It lowers high blood pressure.
2. ***To heal wounds and sores***—Cut fresh tomato into slices. A slice is placed over the wound and tied with adhesive tape. Repeat it for 3 to 4 days. It will heal the wounds.
3. ***To dissolve the fat***—Take one glass juice of fresh tomato fruit once in a day. It usually helps dissolve the fat in body. Thus, hardening of arteries is prevented.
4. ***To relieve diarrhoea***—Cut fine slices of tomato, and dry in oven. Make a powder. Place 2 or 3 spoonfuls of powder in a cup, mix water and take twice a day for diarrhoea.
5. ***To check obesity***—One or two ripe tomatoes taken early morning without breakfast ensures safe weight reduction.

2

CONDIMENTS

1. Asafoetida (Hing)

Botanical name : *Ferula asafoetida* L.

Family : Apiaceae Umbelliferae

Sanskrit name : Hingu

Plant part used : Dry latex obtained from root.

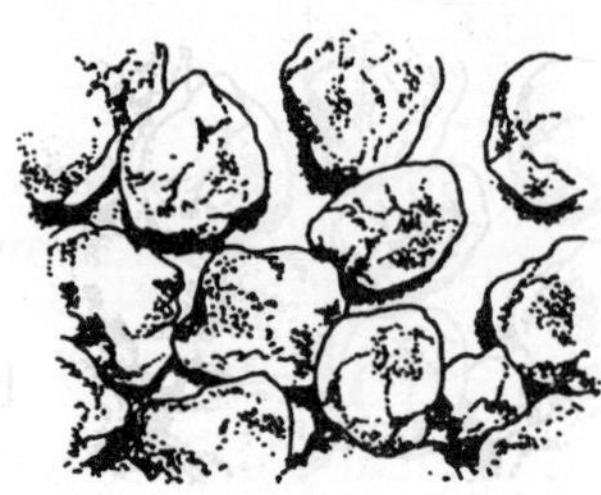

Identification

It is a perennial odourous herb with carrot-shaped root. Leaves pinnately decompound with large sheaths. Flowers smaller, yellow in umbels.

Distribution

It is a native of Mediterranean region from where it spread to Central Asia. Now it is grown in Iran, Afghanistan and Kashmir (India).

Chemical Composition

Asafoetida contains 40-64% resin (asaresinotannol, ferulic acid and umbelliferone), 25% gum, 10-17% volatile oil and 1.5-10% ash.

Medicinal Uses

1. ***To cure intestinal ailments***—Mix equal amounts of asafoetida, black pepper and dry ginger. Prepare soft mixture. Take one spoonful with water three times a day.

2. ***To have relief from burning***—Dissolve asafoetida in water. Apply it over the burnt part of body. Repeat four to five times a day. This will give relief without causing blisters.

3. ***To check toothache***—Warm small part of asafoetida and place it in the cavity of tooth. The pain due to worms will be checked.

4. ***To cure jaundice***—Dissolve a small part of asafoetida in water. Apply it to both eyes twice a day.

5. ***To treat hoarseness***—Take a small part of asafoetida with water twice a day.

6. ***To neutralise the opium poison***—Take asafoetida with water. It will neutralise the effect of opium immediately.

7. ***To cure stomachache***—Dissolve asafoetida in water to prepare a paste. Place it all over the abdomen.

8. ***To treat dilenium***—Dissolve asafoetida in water and place it on palm, sole and nails of hands and feet.

9. ***To cure pinworm disease***—Dissolve asafoetida in water. Place it in anus with the help of cotton. It will give relief in itching of the anus.

10. ***To act as digestant***—Hing and lemon prepation is a good digestant. Seedless lemon pieces mixed with small amount of hing and black salt, left in sun for a week or so, and when rind of lemon becomes soft, it should be taken with meals.

2. Bishop's Weed (Ajwain)

Botanical name : *Trachyspermum ammi* (L.) Sprague

Family : Apiaceae Umbelliferae

Sanskrit name : Ugragandha

Plant part used : Fruits and seeds

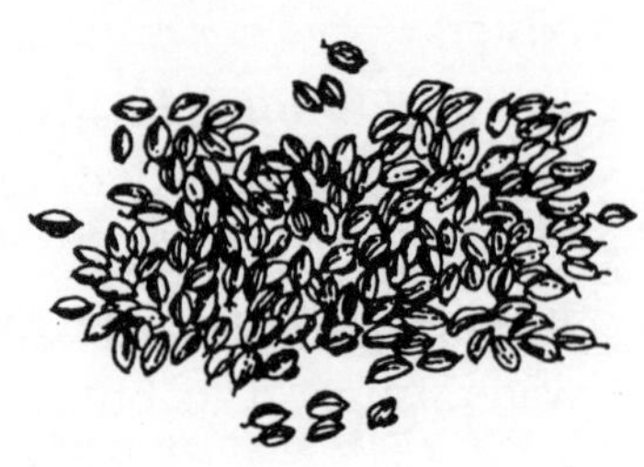

Identification

Erect annual herb up to 1 metre tall. Leaves 2-3 pinnate. Flowers white, in compound umbels. Fruits ovoid and muricate.

Distribution

It is a native of Mediterranean region. It is cultivated in Egypt, Iran, Afghanistan and India. In India, it is grown in W. Bengal, Punjab and other states.

Chemical Composition

The seeds contain 4.8% moisture, 7.1% protein, 7.9% fat, 48.2% carbohydrates, 4.1% mineral matter and 25.0% fibre. They also contain vitamins A, B_1, B_2 and C.

Medicinal Uses

1. ***To cure intestinal ailments***—Make a powder of seeds. Take two spoonfuls of it with warm water in the morning and evening a day.
2. ***To cure cough and cold***—Place three spoonfuls of seeds in water. Boil till water reduces to half. Strain it. Take the juice in the night just before sleep.
3. ***To kill worms in intestine***—Make a powder of seeds. Mix two spoonfuls of powder with black salt in equal amount and take in the night with water.
4. ***To treat gout***—Make a powder of seeds and take two or three spoonfuls with warm milk three times a day.

5. ***To cure dropsy***—Place the seeds in urine of calf and let them dry. Take them three times a day. Dropsy will be cured in one month.

6. ***To treat diabetes***—Grind seeds and *gur* in equal amount. Make four pills. Take them at an interval of 3 hours daily for a month.

7. ***To keep kidney pain away***—Make powder of seeds. Take two spoonfuls in the morning and evening with warm milk.

8. ***To treat influenza***—Boil the seeds in water then strain. Take juice at an interval of two hours daily.

9. ***To cure toothache***—Place the seeds and turmeric powder (*Curcuma Longa* L.) in equal amounts in water. Boil and add a piece of alum; then strain. Take the juice in mouth. Keep for some time touching the teeth and then spit. Repeat it five or more times. The ache of tooth will disappear soon.

10. ***To cure asthma***—Place seeds in *chilam* and burn them. Smoke like a cigarette. Repeat twice a day for a week.

11. ***To treat leucorrhoea***—Place 25 gm seeds and 25 gm sugar candy in a mud vessel filled with water. Keep at night and then grind them in the morning. Take it before breakfast daily for 10 days.

12. ***To check indigestion and dyspepsia***—A small amount of Ajwain when used while making fast food preparations ensures proper digestion.

3. Caraway (Kalajira)

Botanical name : *Carum carvi* L.

Family : Apiaceae
Umbelliferae

Sanskrit name : Shyam jiraka

Plant part used : Fruits and seeds

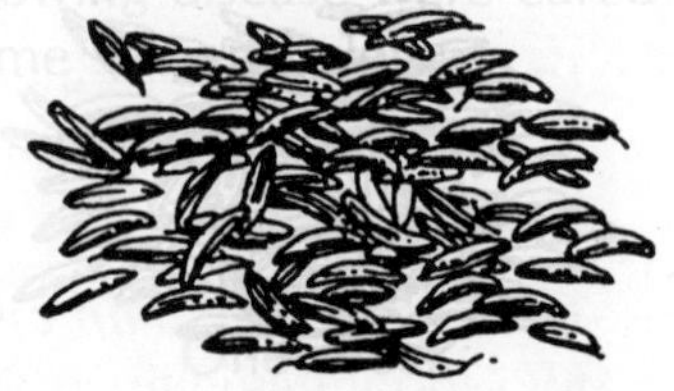

Identification

A biennial herb with tuberous root. Leaves pinnately compound with narrow segments. Flowers white, in dense terminal compound umbels. Fruits oblong, curved, tapering and dark brown in colour.

Distribution

Caraway is indigenous to Europe and Western Asia, now also cultivated in Holland, Russia, Poland, Bulgaria, Syria, Morocco, Turkey, India and England. In India, cultivation is undertaken in Kashmir, Kumaon, Garhwal and Chamba.

Chemical Composition

The caraway seeds contain 4.5% moisture, 7.6% protein, 8.8% fat, 50.2% carbohydrates, 3.7% mineral matter and 25.2% fibre. They also contain vitamins A, B_1, B_2, and C.

Medicinal Uses

1. ***To cure piles***—Mix seeds with sugar candy in equal amount. Make a powder. Take half spoonful of powder with water in the morning and evening.

2. ***To treat dysentery***—Make a powder of the seeds. Mix one spoonful of the powder and one cup of curd. Take it two times a day.

3. ***To relieve gas***—Roasted caraway seed when powdered and mixed with curd and black salt helps check gas formation.

4. Celery (Ajmud)

Botanical name : *Apium graveolens* L.

Family : Apiaceae Umbelliferae

Sanskrit name : Ajmoda

Plant part used : Fruits and seeds

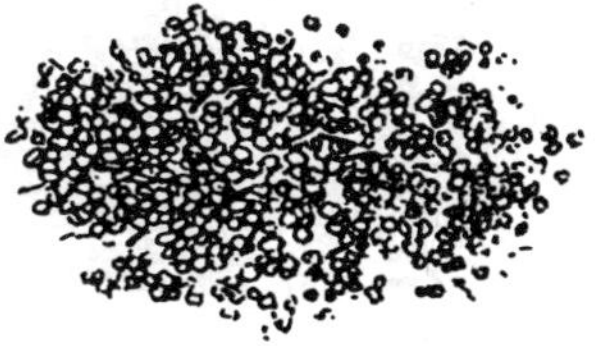

Identification

Perennial herb with dimorphic leaves. Radical leaves pinnate and cauline 3-partite. Flowers small, in leaf-opposed umbels.

Distribution

A native of Europe, now cultivated in France, India and USA. In India, mainly grows in north-west Himalayas, Punjab and UP.

Chemical Composition

The celery seeds contain 5.1% moisture, 18.1% protein, 22.8% fat, 40.9% carbohydrates, 10.2% mineral matter, 2.9% crude fibre and vitamins B_1, B_2, C and A.

Medicinal Uses

1. ***To control body pain***—Take celery seeds and place in mustard oil. Simmer and rub warm mixture on pain sites.
2. ***To cure stomachache***—Make powder of seeds and mix black salt. Take it thrice a day.
3. ***To stop vomiting***—Make powder of seeds and cloves and then mix with honey. Take the mixture to stop vomiting.
4. ***To treat toothache***—Make powder of the seeds. Place it on the site of ache. Rub it gently over teeth and gum. The ache will disappear soon.
5. ***To keep body warm***—Take a few seeds with cold water early in the morning. It will keep cold away.
6. ***To reduce hypertension***—Make powder of seeds and mix with honey. Take thrice a day for a week. Strengthens frayed nerves.

5. Coriander (Dhania)

Botanical name : *Coriandrum sativum* L.

Family : Apiaceae Umbelliferae

Sanskrit name : Dhanyaka

Plant part used : Fruit and seeds

Identification

A small aromatic, annual herb–leaves decompound. Flowers puple or white, in compound umbels. Fruits subglobose, ribbed, yellowish-brown.

Distribution

It is a native of Mediterranean region. It is now cultivated in India, Morocco, Russia, Hungary, Poland, Guatemala, Argentina and the USA. In India, it is grown in Andhra Pradesh, Maharashtra, Tamil Nadu, Punjab, U.P., Assam and M.P.

Chemical Composition

On an average, seeds contain 6.3% moisture, 1.3% protein, 19.6% fat, 24.0% carbohydrates, 5.3% mineral matter, 31.5% crude fibre, and vitamins B_1, B_2, C and A. The pleasant aroma and taste of fruit is due to the presence of an essential oil.

Medicinal Uses

1. ***To neutralise the purging-nut poison***—If one has taken seeds of purging-nut (*Jatropha curcas*) and is suffering from dysentery, give him one spoonful of powder of coriander seeds in curd two or three times a day.
2. ***To relieve inflamed eyes***—Place some seeds in thin cloth and tie forming a bag. Dip it in water and then place gently over the eyes.
3. ***To keep acidity away***—Mix seeds and dry ginger in equal amount. Boil them in water till the water becomes half. Add honey in it and take this mixture twice a day for two weeks.

4. ***To lower high blood pressure***—Take coriander seeds, root of sarpgandha (*Rauwolfia serpentina*) and sugar candy in equal amount. Mix them and make powder. Take two spoonfuls with cold water twice a day.
5. ***To ensure proper sleep***—Take small amount of grinded *Dhania,* say 100 gms, and dip it into a cup of water for a whole day. Take out the water & drink it just before going to bed (there should be a gap of one hour between night meal & taking this water).
6. ***To relieve gas formation***—It is a good remedy to check gas formation. Nearly powdered *Dhania* and *Mishri* pieces, mixed to improve taste, should be taken 3/4 times a day casually.

6. Cumin (Jira)

Botanical name : *Cuminum cyminum* L.

Family : Apiaceae Umbelliferae

Sanskrit name : Jiraka

Plant part used : Fruits and seeds

Identification

A slender, glabrous annual herb. Leaves dissected into filiform segments. Flowers white, in compound umbels. Fruits cylindric.

Distribution

A native of eastern Mediterranean region, it is now cultivated in Iran, India, Morocco, China, Indonesia, Egypt and Argentina. In India, it is grown in U.P., Punjab, Rajasthan, Gujarat and Tamil Nadu.

Chemical Composition

The cumin seeds contain 6.2% moisture, 17.7% protein, 23.8% fat, 35.5% carbohydrates, 7.7% mineral matter, 9.1% crude fibre and vitamins B_1, B_2, C and A.

Medicinal Uses

1. ***To cure stomachache***—Make powder of the cumin seeds and mix honey in equal amount. Lick it slowly.
2. ***To stop dysentery***—Take a cup of curd and mix one spoonful of seed powder and four spoonfuls of water. Take it four times a day at an interval of three hours.
3. ***To cure diarrhoea***—Mix seed powder with curd and take it three times a day.
4. ***To treat dyspepsia***—Mix powder of seeds with *gur* and take in the morning and evening.

5. ***To cure menorrhagia***—Take powder of seeds and sugar candy in equal amounts and then mix them in *ghee*. Take it twice a day.

6. ***To stop vomiting***—Place cumin seeds and common salt in lemon juice. Make a mixture. Take it to stop vomiting.

7. ***To cure anuresis***—Take cumin seeds and sugar candy in equal amounts. Make powder. Take one spoonful with cold water. It will give relief in urination. Repeat it after an interval of four hours.

8. ***To neutralise the spider poison***—Make paste of cumin seeds and dry ginger with water. Apply the paste on the affected part of body.

7. Fennel (Saunf)

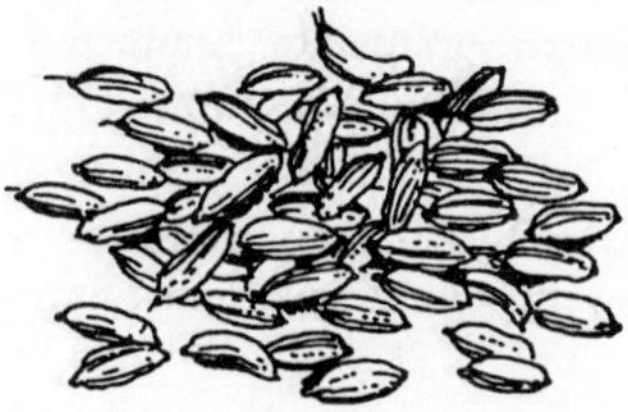

Botanical name : *Foeniculum vulgare* Mill.

Family : Apiaceae Umbelliferae

Sanskrit name : Madhurika

Plant part used : Fruits and seeds

Identification

Erect, glabrous, aromatic herb. Leaves 2 to 4 pinnate, segments thread like. Flowers yellow, in compound umbels. Fruits oblong, pale greenish-yellow.

Distribution

It is a native of southern Europe and the Mediterranean region. It is now grown in India, Russia, Hungary, Italy, Germany, Japan, Argentina and the U.S.A. In India, it is grown in Maharashtra, Gujarat, U.P., Karnataka, Punjab and Rajasthan.

Chemical Composition

Seeds of fennel have essential oil content, varying from 0.7-6.0%. Bitter fennel oil contains about 50-60% of anethole. The sharp flavor of the oil is due to the presence of fenchone.

Medicinal Uses

1. ***To keep digestion fit***—Fry fennel seeds and then mix black salt in equal amount. Take a spoonful in morning and evening. It will remove constipation.
2. ***To have urination cleared***—Prepare a juice of fennel seeds. Place a few drops in a *batasha* and then take two times a day. It will remove the feeling of difficulty and pain during urination.
3. ***To make pregnancy possible***—Make a powder of seeds and mix with cow's *ghee*. Take 5 grams of the mixture daily for three months.

4. ***To cure dyspepsia***–Take fennel seeds after meal and chew them slowly.
5. ***To treat dysentery***–Make a powder of seeds and mix with rind of Bael fruit (*Aegle marmelos*) in equal amount. Take a spoonful with curd thrice a day.
6. ***To heal pimples and boils***–Place 50 gm of funnel seeds in mud pitcher for a night and take a bath in the morning. It will heal pimples and boils present in any part of the body during summer.
7. ***To make eyesight strong***–Mix fennel seeds and sugar candy in equal amounts and then prepare a powder. Take two spoonfuls of the powder with fresh water before going to bed. It will improve the eyesight and will check the formation of cataract.
8. ***To make child's teething easy***–Boil fennel seeds in water and then strain. Mix a spoonful of it in milk. Give it to a child thrice a day. The child will not feel indigestion, dysentery and pain during the teething period.
9. ***To check body's heat/acidity***–One glass of sounf sharbat in the morning keeps the whole day cool. Saunf 100 gms in a cup of water whole night and in the morning its paste in prepared, this paste is dissolved in a glass of water & sugar. It is taken without eating anything.

8. Fenugreek (Methi)

Botanical name : *Trigonella foenum-graecum* L.
Family : Apiaceae Papilionaceae
Sanskrit name : Methika
Plant part used : Seeds

Identification

Erect, annual herb. Leaves pinnately 3-foliate, toothed. Flowers white or pale-yellow, axillary. Pods sickle-shaped. Seeds yellowish-brown, deeply furrowed.

Distribution

It is a native of eastern Europe and Ethiopia. It is now cultivated in Hungary, Poland, Russia, China, India, Argentina, Brazil and the U.S.A. In India, it is grown in U.P., Punjab, M.P., Maharashtra etc.

Chemical Composition

Fenugreek seeds contain 8.6% moisture, 35.7% carbohydrates, 10.4% protein, 15.9% fats, 20.1% fibre, 6.5% mineral matter and vitamins B_1, B_2, C and A.

Medicinal Uses

1. ***To cure diabetes***—Place two spoonfuls of fenugreek seeds in water for a night. Take them in the morning before breakfast. It will certainly reduce the sugar level in blood as well as in urine within a couple of months.
2. ***To control blood pressure***—Mix fenugreek seeds and dill seeds (*Anethum sowa*) in equal amounts and then make their powder. Take two spoonfuls in the morning and evening with fresh water. It will maintain blood pressure normal.
3. ***To reduce cholesterol***—Place seeds in water at night. Take soaked seeds orally with water twice a day. The serum cholesterol level will be reduced.

4. ***To cure hay fever***—Place seeds in cold water for 5 hours and then boil for two minutes. Take one cup a day.
5. ***To stop bleeding***—Boil fenugreek seeds in milk. Cool and then strain. Mix sugar candy and then take the mixture. Bleeding from any part of the body stops.
6. ***To treat asthma***—Boil the seeds and then crush them into a paste. Mix honey, take it twice a day for one month.
7. ***To keep joints fit***—Prepare a powder of seeds. Dissolve 5 gm of powdered seeds in water and take twice a day regularly. Chances of pain in any joint of body will not occur even in older days.
8. ***To check respiratory diseases***—Tea of seeds will help in bronchitis, influenza, sinusitis, pneumonia etc.

9. Red Pepper [Lal Mirch (Chilli)]

Botanical name : *Capsicum annuum* Linn.

Family : Solanaceae

Sanskrit name :

Plant part used : Dried ripe fruits

Identification

A small, bushy annual herb. Flowers solitary axillary white. Fruits green, turn red when ripe.

Distribution

It is a native of tropical America and the West Indies. Chillies are now cultivated in Africa, India, Japan, Turkey, Mexico, the U.S.A. and West Indies. In India, Karnataka, Orissa, Maharastra, Rajasthan and Tamil Nadu.

Chemical Composition

On an average, dried chillies contain 10% moisture, 15.9% protein, 6.2% fats, 31.6% carbohydrates, 30.2% fibres and 6.1% ash. They also contain vitamins (riboflavin, niacin and ascorbic acid). The pungency is due to a crystalline phenolic substance known as capsaicin.

Medicinal Uses

1. ***To lower cholesterol level***—Mix seeds of chillies, drops of lemon juice and tomato juice. Consume it regularly twice a day. It will lower the cholesterol level.

2. ***To treat dog bite***—Grind red peppers in water to prepare a paste. Apply it directly on the bites. It will first check the bleeding and then will heal the injured parts.

3. ***To prevent blood clots***—Consume red peppers in your diet regularly. The chances of blood clot problems are prevented.

4. ***To cure swollen and painful joints***—Warm red peppers and mix them to the melted vaseline. Cool it and store. Apply it once daily to the sprains, bruises and swollen places.

5. ***To heal the ulcer***—Consume red peppers in your diet regularly. It stimulates the intestinal mucosal cells to release more slimy mucous. Such mucous passes into the intestine touching ulcers. In the course of time, the ulcer gets healed up.

6. ***To keep body warm in winter***—Place two or more chillies in your socks and in gloves when you are out in winter. Chillies will be helpful in providing warmth to the body during the winter.

Warning

Those, who are having low sugar level in blood, should avoid taking chillies.

10. Turmeric (Haldi)

Botanical name : *Curcuma longa* L.

Family : Zingiberaceae

Sanskrit name : Haridra

Plant part used : Rhizome

Identification

A tall aromatic perennial herb. Rhizome large, ovoid, yellow or orange in side. Leaves large, broad, lanceolate. Flowers pale-yellow, in spikes, covered by pink bracts. Turmeric is a sterile triploid.

Distribution

A native of south-eastern Asia is known to India since ancient times. It is now cultivated in India, China, Indonesia and Taiwan. In India, it is grown in A.P., Maharashtra, Orissa, Tamil Nadu, Karnataka and Kerala.

Chemical Composition

Dry turmeric contains 5.8% moisture, 8.6% protein, 8.9% fat, 63.0% carbohydrates, 6.9% fibre, 6.8% mineral matter and vitamins A, B_1, B_2, C. It also contains calcium, phosphorus, iron, sodium and potassium.

Medicinal Uses

1. ***To check gastric problem***—Mix turmeric powder and common salt in equal amounts. Take it two spoonfuls with warm water two times a day. It will give relief in gas formation as well as in indigestion discomforts.
2. ***To cure bronchitis***—Take one spoonful turmeric powder with warm water three times a day. It will make phlegm melt.
3. ***To give protection against cancer***—Add two spoonfuls turmeric powder in a cup of water. Stir and then take it

regularly twice a day. It has active components (curcumol and curdione), which have strong cytotoxic effects against certain forms of cancer.

4. ***To relieve pain and itching of skin***—Mix turmeric powder with the lime juice (*Citrus limon*) and a little water to make a smooth paste. Put it directly on to herpes lesions, eczema, psoriasis, pimples and even leprosy sores.

5. ***To stop bleeding during pregnancy***—Add two spoonfuls of turmeric powder in boiling water. Take one cup at early pregnancy bleeding. Repeat it as long as needed to stop bleeding.

6. ***To relieve sprains and internal injuries***—Add one spoonful turmeric powder in two cups of milk. Simmer and then let it be cool. Take one cup regularly in the morning and evening.

7. ***To treat acne and black spots at face***—Mix equal amount of turmeric powder and gram flour in curd. Make a paste. Apply it over the face for acne and black spots.

8. ***To treat piles***—Take one spoonful turmeric powder with water in the morning and evening.

9. ***To stop hiccup***—Place 4 gm turmeric powder in a *chilam* and then burn it. Smoke like a cigarette. It will stop hiccup immediately.

10. ***To cure diabetes***—Mix turmeric powder and honey in equal amounts. Lick it.

11. ***To treat cough and cold***—Add one spoonful turmeric powder in one cup milk. Simmer and then add sugar. Take it in the morning and evening.

12. ***To relieve joints pain and backache***—Unripe turmeric is made into paste and boiled in milk in 1:5 proportion and a kind of Halua or semi solid paste is prepared. Now, sugar is added as per the taste. It is taken a teaspoonful in the morning and evening.

3

SPICES

1. Black Pepper (Kali Mirch)

Botanical name : *Piper nigrum* L.

Family : Piperaceae

Sanskrit name : Maricha

Plant part used : Dried unripe fruits

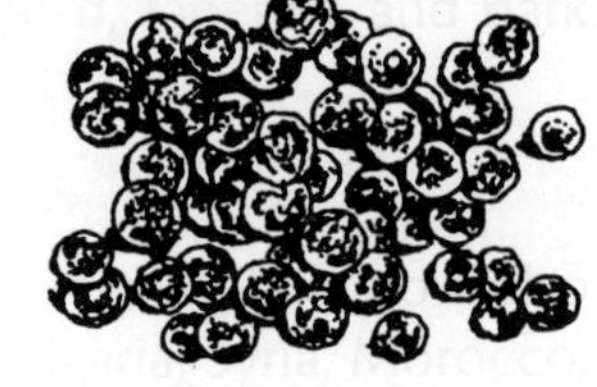

Identification

Perennial vine. The vine has dimorphic branching. Leaves ovate with pungent taste. Flowers small, white, in dense spike, partially enclosed by a fleshy bract. Fruit drupe, bright red, which becomes black and wrinkled.

Distribution

Indigenous to the damp forests of the Malabar coast of south-western India. It is now cultivated in Indonesia, Philippines, Thailand, Malaysia, tropical Africa and India. In India, it is grown in Kerala, Karnataka, Tamil Nadu etc.

Chemical Composition

On an average, black pepper contains 8.8-14.4% moisture, 38.0-49.0% carbohydrates, 8.0-18.0% crude fibres, 3.0-6.7% total ash, 2.5-3.6% total nitrogen, 3.8-8.9% piparine and pipasine. The aromatic odour is due to the presence of volatile oil.

Medicinal Uses

1. ***To make water pure***—Boil water and place two spoonfuls of black pepper and allow to cool. Strain and then take it.

2. ***To treat hoarseness and sore throat***—Make a powder of the black pepper and place it in water. Warm it. Gargle four times a day.
3. ***To cure gonorrhoea***—Mix black pepper and chueb piper (*Piper cubeca*) in equal amounts. Make a powder and then take three times a day with fresh water.
4. ***To make sneezing easy***—Make powder of black pepper. Take it inside the nostrils. Breathe gently. It will help sneeze. The headache due to cold will disappear soon.
5. ***To reduce acidity***—Make a powder of black pepper and mix honey and *ghee*. Take it two times a day regularly for one month.
6. ***To cure pimples***—Grind black pepper with water to prepare a paste. Apply it over the eyelid's pimples three times a day.
7. ***To treat hemicrania***—Make a paste of black pepper. Apply it in the eye opposite to the site of pain on forehead.
8. ***To eliminate hay fever***—Crush some leaves of holy basil (*Ocimum sanctum*) and black pepper and then mix them in tea. Take it three times a day. It will relieve the fever also.
9. ***To cure stammering***—Mix almond without seed coat (*Prunus amygdalus*) and black pepper in equal amounts. Grind and then add sugar candy. Lick the mixture two times a day.
10. ***To overcome mental fatique***—Grind black pepper and sugar candy and then mix butter. Take this mixture in the morning for one month.
11. ***To treat colic pain***—Boil black pepper in milk. When milk reduces to half then cool. Take it three times a day.
12. ***To relieve calf muscle pain***—Four/five seeds of black pepper to be chewed at the bed time to get relief from this pain.

2. Cinnamon (Dal Chini)

Botanical name : *Cinnamomum Verun J.S. Presl Syn. C. zeylanicum* Garc

Family : Lauraceae

Sanskrit name : Tamal patra

Plant part used : Dried inner bark of stem

Identification

A small evergreen tree. Leaves large, ovate, leathery. Flowers minute, yellow, in large, hairy clusters. Fruits oblong, dark and purple.

Distribution

It is a native of Sri Lanka. It is now cultivated in Sri Lanka, India, Malaysia, Indonesia, Kenya, China, West Indies and Seychelles.

Chemical Composition

The bark contains 0.5 to 1.5% essential oil. Its chief constituent is cinnamic aldehyde (60-75%). Cinnamon leaf oil contains 70-95% eugenol.

Medicinal Uses

1. ***To cure dysentery***—Make a powder of cinnamon. Take 2 gm twice a day with water.
2. ***To treat stammering***—Take a piece of cinnamon in mouth and chew it thoroughly before swallowing.
3. ***To keep cold and flu away***—Take cinnamon and Bishop's seed (*Trachyspermum ammi*) in equal amounts. Give slow boil for three minutes in water. Strain and then take half cup in the morning and half cup in the evening. It cures fever and congestion.
4. ***To make sexual rejuvenation***—Take 3 gm cinnamon with warm milk daily at night before sleep. It will increase the sperm count and will also promote sexual stimulation.

3. Clove (Laung)

Botanical name : *Eugenia caryophyllus Bull & Hars Syzygium aromaticum* (Merr. & Perry)

Family : Myrtaceae

Sanskrit name : Lavanga

Plant part used : Dried floral buds

Identification

A small evergreen tree. Leaves opposite, glabrous, dotted with oil glands. Flowers crimson, in terminal panicled cymes. Fruits purple drupe.

Distribution

It is indigenous to the Moluccas. It was introduced in India in 1800 A.D. by the East India Company. It is now grown in Tanzania, Pemba Islands, Madagascar, Indonesia, Sri Lanka, Malaysia and Haiti. In India, it is mainly grown in Nilgiri, Tanbasi Hills and Kanyakumari (Tamil Nadu) and Kottayam and Quilon (Kerala).

Chemical Composition

On an average, cloves contain 5.4% moisture, 6.5% protein, 15.3% fat, 10.9% crude fibre, 57.8% carbohydrates, 5.0% mineral matter and vitamins B_1, B_2, C and A. Cloves also contain 13.6% essential oil (Eugenol and caryophylline).

Medicinal Uses

1. ***To stop bad breath***—Take two cups of hot water and place three cloves. Leave it for 30 minutes and then filter. Gargle twice a day for mouth wash.
2. ***To check alcohol carvings***—Put two cloves in mouth then suck slowly. Be careful not to chew them. The carvings are effectively checked for the time being.

3. ***To curb vomiting in pregnant woman***—Boil 3 gm cloves in 3 kg water till water becomes half. Sip it slowly to check vomiting.
4. ***To cure cough***—Roast 3 cloves and mix them in *gur*. Lick it to cure cough.
5. ***To treat intestinal disorders***—Take an apple and remove its fruit wall. Fix sufficient cloves entering their lower parts inside the fruit. Put such fruit for 40 days in a protected place. Take all the cloves out of the fruit and store them. After meal take one clove and suck slowly. It will give relief in all the ailments concerned with stomach.
6. ***To give relief in cold***—Boil 3 cloves in water and then filter. Suck water through nostrils.
7. ***To remove pimple***—Rub clove with water on a stone. Put the paste over eyelid's pimple. It will destroy the pimple immediately.
8. ***To cure toothache***—Take clove oil or clove paste in cotton. Place such cotton over the suffering tooth. It will give relief in the pain.
9. ***To make sore throat better***—Place two cloves in a betel leaf *(Pipper betle L.)*. Take it twice a day.

4. Large Cardamom (Bari Ilaichi)

Botanical name : *Amomum sabulatum Roxb.*

Family : Zingiberaceae

Sanskrit name : Brihadaela

Plant part used : Seeds

Identification

Perennial herb with underground rhizome. Leaves large, lanceolate with leaf-sheathing. Flowers borne on separated elongated stalk. The fruits are larger.

Distribution

A native of Nepal. Now it is cultivated in swampy places along the sides of mountain streams in Nepal and India. In India, it is cultivated in W. Bengal, Sikkim and Assam.

Chemical Composition

Average seed has 9.1% moisture, 8.7% volatile oil, 5.0% total ash, 12.1% crude fibre, 10.0% crude protein, 45.0% carbohydrates, 1.7% minerals and vitamins B_1, B_2, C & A.

Medicinal Uses

1. ***To cure anuresis***—Powder it and boil in milk. When milk becomes half, cool it. Add sugar candy. Take it four times a day for all kinds of urinary ailments.
2. ***To heal liver ailments***—Make a powder of seeds. Take it three times a day with cold water.
3. ***To keep headache away***—Take husks and grind them in water to make a paste. Apply this paste over the forehead.
4. ***To treat leucorrhoea***—Take seeds and *Majuphal* (*Cuercus infectoria Oliv.*) in equal amounts. Make a powder and add sugar candy. Take it twice a day with fresh water.
5. ***To stop hiccup***—Crush large cardamom and place in water. Boil it till water becomes half. Keep it to become cool. Take it slowly. Hiccup will be stopped immediately.

5. Long Pepper (Peepar)

Botanical name : *Piper longum* L.

Family : Piperaceae

Sanskrit name : Pippalee

Plant part used : Dried unripe fruit (root as a piplimool)

Identification

A small trailing or climbing aromatic plant with perennial woody roots. Lower leaves broad, ovate and upper leaves oblong-ovate. Fruits small, ovoid, blackish-green.

Distribution

It is a native of India and Sri Lanka. It is cultivated in Sri Lanka, India, Singapore, Malaysia and Philippines. In India, it is common in Western Ghats, Assam, Nagaland and lower hills of W. Bengal.

Chemical Composition

Long pepper contains 11.7% moisture, 41% carbohydrates, 8.3% crude fibre, 4.1% total ash, and vitamins B_1, B_2, C and A. Biting taste is due to an alkaloid, paparine.

Medicinal Uses

1. ***To cure epilepsy***—Make a powder of fruits. Take one spoonful twice a day with water.
2. ***To treat chronic bronchitis***—Boil fruits in water. When water becomes half then strain. Take the juice twice a day for one month.
3. ***To treat goitre***—Make powder of seeds and mix it with honey in equal amount. Lick it twice a day.
4. ***To keep cough away***—Mix powder of fruit with honey. Take it at night before sleep.
5. ***To keep spleen fit***—Make a powder of the fruit and give one spoonful with cow's milk once a day.

6. Javitri [Aril (Nutmeg)], Jaiphal (Seed)

Botanical name : *Myristica fragrans* Houtt

Family : Myristicaceae

Sanskrit name : Jatiphal

Plant part used : Seed (Nutmeg) and aril (Mace)

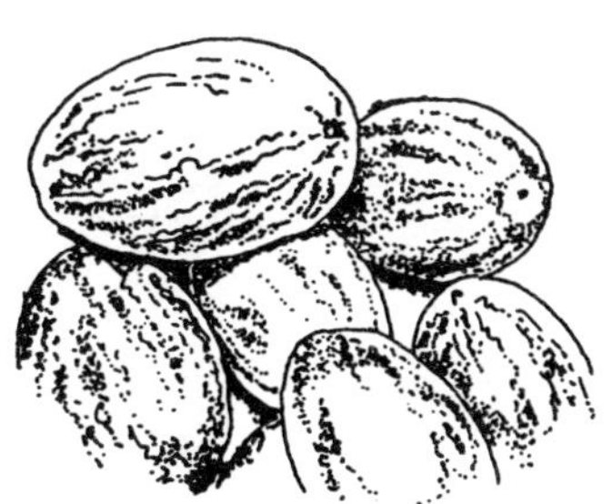

Identification

It is an evergreen tree with the height of 30-60 feet. Leaves dark green. It is dioecious with small pale-yellow flowers. Fruits golden-yellow in colour when ripe. When fruits become dry, the husk splits open releasing shiny brown seed (Nutmeg) covered with a bright scarlet aril (Mace).

Distribution

It is a native of Moluccas Islands. In India, it is grown in the Nilgiris, Kerala, Karnataka and W. Bengal.

Chemical Composition

Nutmeg consists of 14.3%, moisture, 7.5% protein, 28.6% carbohydrates, 11.6% fibre, 1.7% mineral matter, 6.16% nutmeg oil, 2.5% pentosans, 1.5% furfural, 0.6% pectin and vitamins B_1, B_2, C and A.

Medicinal Uses

1. ***To cure dysentery***—Grind seeds in water and take twice a day with the water of curd.
2. ***To treat acne***—Mix seeds in milk to prepare a paste. Apply it over the acne and pimples before sleep for one month.
3. ***To keep epilepsy away***—Take 21 seeds and make a rosary. Place it around the neck of patient. It will keep epilepsy away.

4. ***To cure insomnia***—Prepare a paste of seeds in *ghee*. Apply it over the eyelids. The patient will get a sound sleep.

5. ***To cure arthritis***—Make a powder of seeds and mix it with mustard oil (*Brassica campestris*). Rub it over the joints. The pain of joints will be cured within a month.

6. ***To treat headache***—Prepare a paste by rubbing seeds on a stone. Apply it over the nostrils and forehead.

7. ***To treat lumbago***—Make a powder of seeds and mix it with wine to prepare a paste. Apply it over the site of pain in loin.

8. ***To treat cholera***—Roast seeds and mix with *gur*. Make pills of small size. Take a pill at an interval of 10 minutes.

Warning

Excessive doses of nutmeg taken orally will produce narcotic effect, causing delirium and epileptic convulsions after 1-6 hours.

7. Small Cardamom (Chhoti Ilaichi)

Botanical name : *Elettaria cardamomum (L.)* Maton

Family : Zingiberaceae

Sanskrit name : Ela

Plant part used : Fruit and seeds.

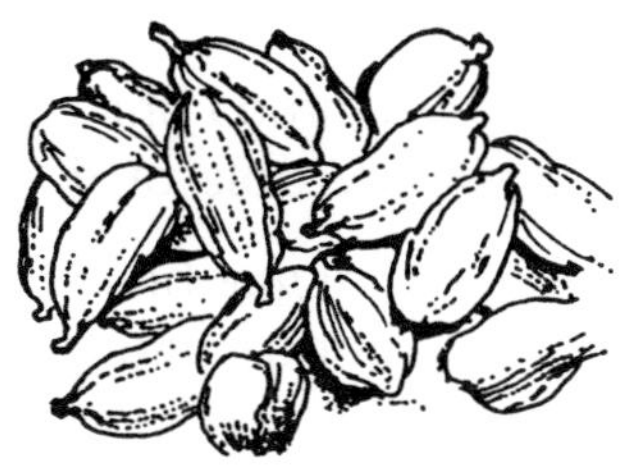

Identification

A tall perennial herb with several erect leafy shoots and underground rhizome. Leaves lanceolate, dark green with leaf sheath. Flowers on long panicles. Fruit is a trilocular capsule, white, oblong, ovoid, with 10-15 seeds.

Distribution

It is a native of South India and Sri Lanka. It is now cultivated in India, Sri Lanka, Guatemala, Thailand, Laos, Vietnam, Costa Rica, El Salvador and Tanzania. In India, it is grown in Kerala, Karnataka and Tamil Nadu.

Chemical Composition

Cardamom seeds contain 7-10% moisture, 5.0-10.0% volatile oil, 3.2-6.7% total ash, 6.9 to 13.0% crude fibre, 7.0-14.0% protein, 38.8 to 50.1% carbohydrates and vitamins B_1, B_2, C and A. The seeds have a characteristic aroma due to cineol, terpineol, turpinene, sabinene and limonene.

Medicinal Uses

1. ***To cure headache***—Take seeds and make a powder. Place the powder inside the nostrils and then breathe gently. After sneezing, the pain will disappear.

2. ***To treat cholera***—Take husks and grind them. Boil till water reduces to one fourth. Leave for cooling and then strain. Take half cup several times. It will stop vomiting, thirst and will clear urination.

3. ***To cure spermatorrhoea***—Mix seeds and husk of Isabgul (*Plantago ovata*) in equal amounts. Grind them with fresh fruits of *anola* (*Emblica officinalis*). Make pills. Take one pill in the morning and one in evening with cow's milk.
4. ***To improve eyesight***—Mix seeds and sugar candy in equal amounts. Grind them in the form of powder. Add the powder in pure castor oil and take it twice a day.
5. ***To cure liver disorder***—Make powder of seeds and boil in water. When water reduces to half, cool it, take two times a day.
6. ***To relieve the scorpion sting***—Take seeds in mouth and chew them. Blow in the ear of patient. The pain will disappear immediately.
7. ***To neutralise the poison of Jamalgota***—Make the powder of seeds and add it in curd. Take such curd twice a day for 3 days only. The poison of *Jamalgota* (*Jatropha curcas*) will disappear soon.

8. Tamala (Tejpat)

Botanical name : *Cinnamomum tamala (Spreng)* Nees & Eber

Family : Lauraceae

Sanskrit name : Tamalaka, Tamal patra

Plant part used : Leaves

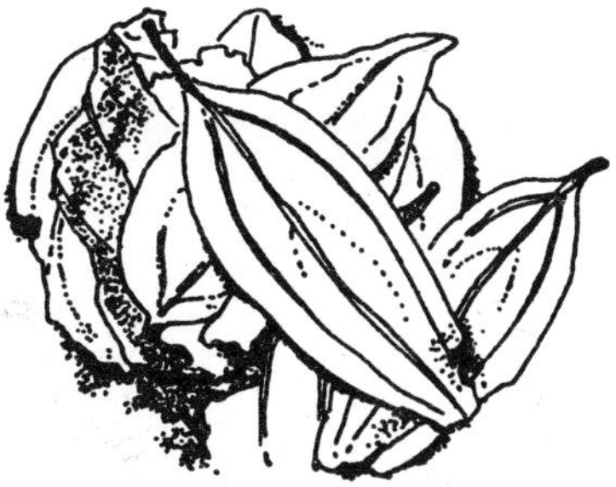

Identification

Evergreen moderate tree. Leaves ovate-oblong, lanceolate. Fruits oval.

Distribution

It is a native of tropical and sub-tropical Himalayas. It is cultivated in Manipur, Tripura, Sikkim, Meghalaya and Nagaland.

Chemical Composition

The dried leaves contain 5.7% moisture, 10.2% protein, 20.1% fat, 15.2% crude fibre, 45% carbohydrates, 6.6% total ash, 3.1% mineral matter, vitamins B_1, B_2, C and A. Leaves contain an essential oil with phellendrene and eugenol.

Medicinal Uses

1. ***To treat gout***—Grind the leaves and make a paste. Apply it over the inflammation of joints twice a day.
2. ***To destroy the kidney stone***—Use the leaves as spice in vegetables, curry or meat. The stones in kidney or in urinary bladder will soon break and pass out through urine.
3. ***To minimise the intestinal gas***—Take leaves regularly in vegetables, curries and meat. It will reduce the possibility of gas formation in intestine.

4

FLAVOUR YIELDING PLANTS

1. Garlic (Lahsun)

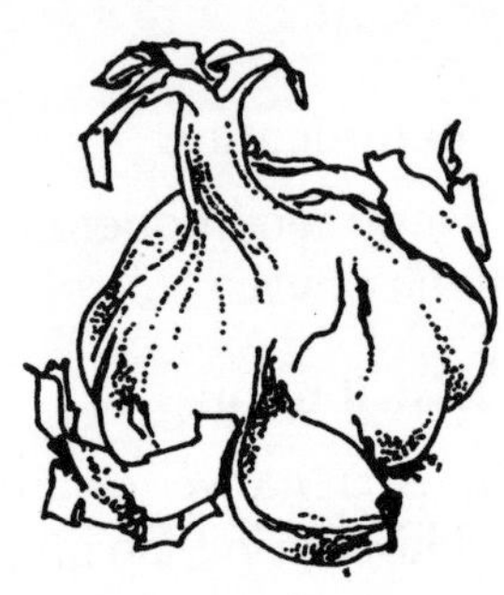

Botanical name : *Allium sativum* L.

Family : Liliaceae

Sanskrit name : Alliaceae, Arishtha

Plant part used : Underground stem called bulb containing many cloves.

Identification

A biennial herb with underground stem called bulb. The bulb has many small bulblets (cloves) enclosed in white or pink envelopes. Leaves flat. Flowers pink, in lax umbels on a long scape.

Distribution

It is a native of Central Asia and eastern Mediterranean region. It is widely grown in India, China, Spain, Egypt, Korea, Argentina, Italy and the U.S.A. In India, it is cultivated throughout the country.

Chemical Composition

On an average, garlic bulbs consist of 62% moisture, 28% carbohydrates, 6.5% proteins, 0.8% fats, 0.9% minerals, 1.1% crude fibres and traces of vitamins B_1, B_2, C and A. Bulbs also possess 1.0% essential oil with sulphur compounds allicin and allisatin.

Medicinal Uses

1. ***To eliminate worms***—Take fresh cut cloves alongwith the diet. After some days the intestinal parasites will get expelled.
2. ***To be helpful in diabetes***—Take two to four cloves with water every morning.
3. ***To increase longevity***—Take freshly cut two or three cloves with the diet every day. It will increase the age.
4. ***To lower serum cholesterol***—Consume two to five freshly cut cloves per day in diet. It will certainly clean the arteries of bad cholesterol. The cholesterol is the main cause for chocking of the flow of blood through the heart. Garlic, therefore, protects against atherosclerosis.
5. ***To cure bacteria-induced diarrhoea***—Crush four cloves, boil them in three cups of water for half an hour. Cool and then take. Take it thrice a day.
6. ***To act as mosquito repellant***—Peel 10 garlic cloves and grind them. Squeeze juice and mix in half cup of olive oil. Keep it for a week. Rub arms, legs, hands, face and neck with it before sleep. It will keep mosquitoes away.
7. ***To treat toothache***—Crush a clove and then place it over the bad tooth. The ache will soon go away.
8. ***To cure chest congestion***—Crush about seven garlic cloves and then place in mustard oil. Boil for about three hours. Leave it to cool after stirring well. Store for use. Rub this ointment on the throat, chest, abdomen and upper portion of the back between the shoulder blades. It will break the phlegm and will make breathing easy.
9. ***To reduce hypertension***—Grind three or four cloves. Squeeze juice and mix in honey in equal amount. Take it in the morning every day. This will help control high blood pressure.
10. ***To treat hysteria***—Peel five to seven cloves and keep them in warm milk for three hours. Take them twice a day.
11. ***To cure paralysis***—Take one clove in the morning with water on first day. Gradually increase the number of cloves

according to the number of days for three weeks. Thus, on 21st day, take 21 cloves. Now reduce one clove each day for three weeks. Thus, on 42nd day, take one clove.

12. ***Aphrodisiac***—Activates prostatic function and increases sex-ability. Four cloves to be chewed daily.
13. ***Skin diseases***—It is a proven dermatitis & antifungal agent. Its juice is rubbed on the affected parts.
14. ***Common cold***—It has preventive role in common cold. Two to four cloves to be taken in the morning.
15. ***Anti-amoebic***—It is a powerful herbal medicine against amoebic dysentery equivalent to metronidazole (Metrogyl).

2. Ginger (Adarakh)

Botanical name : *Zingiber officinale* Rosc.

Family : Zingiberaceae

Sanskrit name : Adrak

Plant part used : Underground fresh rhizome and dry rhizome (Sonth).

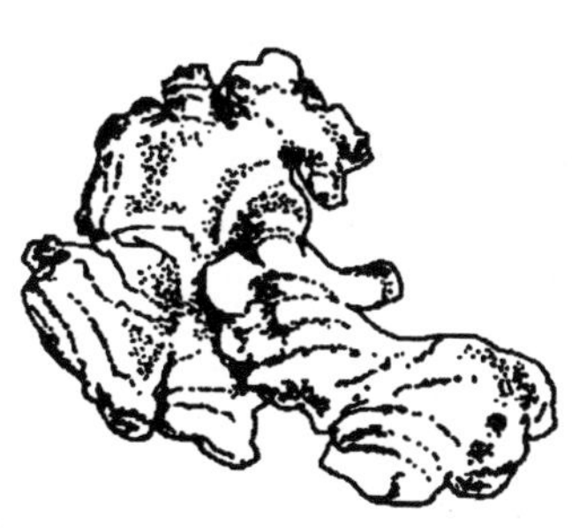

Identification

The plant is an erect perennial herb. The underground rhizome is branched, covered with small-scale leaves. The leafy shoots are annual, erect. The leaves are linear-lanceolate with sheathing bases. The flowers are pale yellow in a dense spike.

Distribution

Ginger is indigenous to South-east Asia. It was introduced in European countries in the 9th century. It is now cultivated in India, Jamaica, China, Japan, Australia, Nigeria, and Taiwan. In India, it is grown in Kerala, Orissa, West Bengal, M.P., Himachal Pradesh, Karnataka and Gujarat.

Chemical Composition

On an average, dry ginger contains 6.8% moisture, 8.6% protein, 6.5% fat, 6.0% crude fibre, 66.5% carbohydrates, 5.5% ash, 1.7% mineral matter and vitamins A, B_1, B_2 and C. The characteristic aroma is due to a pale yellow viscid essential oil (ginger oil), which contains zingiberene, zingiberol, d-camphene and geraniol.

Medicinal Uses

1. ***To eliminate phlegm***—Crush ginger and then add them to 2 cups of boiling water and cover. Steep for 30

minutes. Take one cup while still warm at an interval of three hours.

2. ***To cure dyspepsia***—Cut fresh ginger into small pieces. Add lemon juice and salt. Store the mixture. Take 3 or 4 pieces after a meal.

3. ***To give relief in cough***—Squeeze juice of fresh ginger. Mix one spoonful of juice with one spoonful of honey. Take it thrice a day.

4. ***To stop hiccup***—Boil dry ginger goat's milk. When milk becomes half then cool. Take it to stop hiccup.

5. ***To cure hemicrania***—Make a powder of dry ginger and mix fresh water to prepare a paste. Apply it on the forehead and temporal region.

6. ***To keep nausea away***—Make a powder of dry ginger and add fresh water. Take it twice a day.

7. ***To protect against influenza***—Squeeze juice of fresh ginger and mix it with honey in equal amount. Take it two times a day as preventive cure during the change of season and at the time of viral fever.

8. ***To act as hydrocele remedy***—Squeeze juice of fresh ginger and Mix with one spoonful of honey. Take it in the morning for a month.

9. ***To cure dropsy***—Mix juice of fresh ginger with old *gur* (Molasses). Take it twice a day. The patient should drink goat's milk only.

10. ***To keep eyes healthy***—Burn dry ginger to an ash. Make a fine powder of the ash. Apply it in the eyes before sleep. It will check the eye diseases and will keep eyes healthy.

11. ***To cure bronchitis***—Boil one spoonful of the dry ginger powder in two cups of water. When water becomes half, cool it. Filter and then take two times a day.

12. ***To make delivery easy***—Prepare powder of dry ginger. Take two spoonfuls with warm milk at the time of labour pain.

13. ***Fever***—It is a powerful anti-viral agent and gives relief to much extent as far as viral fever is concerned.
14. ***Sore throat***—It is an effective remedy in sore throat and opens the voice when taken with little salt.
15. ***Aphrodisiac***—It is a potent aphrodisiac when taken with honey and onion juice (ratio 1:2:1).
16. ***To check vomiting***—Mix the juice of ginger and juice of onion in equal 2 spoons of the mixture.
17. ***To treat gum trouble***—Take 5 gm powder of dry ginger (*sonth*) with water.

Warning

The patients suffering from leprosy, jaundice, boils plethora and gonorrhoea should not take ginger especially during the summer and the autumn.

3. Indian Mustard (Rai)

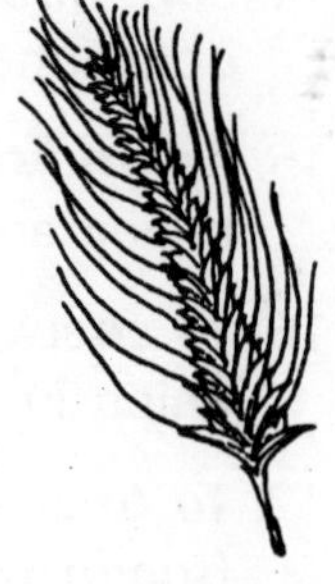

Botanical name : *Brassica juncea* (L.) Czern. & Coss.

Family : Brassicaceae cruciferae

Sanskrit name : Rajika, Tikshnagandha

Plant part used : Seeds

Identification

An erect, much-branched annual herb. The basal leaves stalked, lyrate with large terminal segment. Flowers are small, yellow, in corymbose racemes. The fruit is siliqua. Seeds yellow.

Distribution

It is a native of Africa, especially the Mediterranean region. It is extensively cultivated in Europe, China, Southern Asia and Africa. In India, it is grown in U.P., Punjab, Rajasthan, Assam and M.P.

Chemical Composition

On an average, seeds contain 90.6% moisture, 2.6% protein, 0.4% fat, 4.8% carbohydrate, 1.0% crude fibre, 1.6% ash and vitamin A and C. Seeds yield pale-yellow oil.

Medicinal Uses

1. ***To cure cold***—Grind seeds, sugar and black pepper to form a powder. Take it twice a day with warm water.
2. ***To relieve epilepsy***—Grind seeds as powder. Smell it through nostrils at the time of attack. It will give relief.
3. ***To remove itching***—Grind seeds in cow's urine and mix with clay soil to make a paste. Apply it over the itching places on the body.

4. ***To kill intestinal worms***—Grind seeds and mix with cow's urine. Take two times a day. Worms will be killed and pass through feces.
5. ***To heal wounds***—Grind seeds to powder. Mix the powder with honey. Place it above the wound and tie a clove above it.
6. ***To cure toothache***—Boil seeds and make a soft paste. Apply it over the affected tooth.
7. ***To reduce the phlegm***—Grind seeds to powder. Grind turmeric and fry it. Now mix both powders and store in a bottle. Take powder with honey two times a day.
8. ***To treat ringworm***—Grind seeds to powder. Mix powder with vinegar. Apply it over the ringworm twice a day.
9. ***To control asthma***—Mix powder of seeds, honey and *ghee*. Take this mixture twice a day.
10. ***To improve indigestion***—Make a powder of seeds and mix sugar. Take this mixture twice a day.

4. Mint (Pudina)

Botanical name : *Mentha longifolia* (L.) Huds.

Family : Lamiaceae Labiatae

Sanskrit name : Podeenaka

Plant part used : Whole plant and leaves

Identification

A branched, erect, aromatic, perennial herb. Leaves sessile, ovate-lanceolate, serrate. Flowers white in spikes.

Distribution

It is a native of Europe and Asia. It is cultivated in France, India, China, Indonesia and Germany. In India, it is grown in Kashmir, Punjab, Maharashtra, Uttar Pradesh and Madhya Pradesh.

Chemical Composition

Green leaves contain 92% moisture, 2.9% carbohydrates, 2% proteins, 0.6% ‘ats, 0.5% fibres and 1.9% minerals. They also contain vitamins A, B_1 and C. Leaves yield essential oil, which contains d-menthol, menthone and limonine.

Medicinal Uses

1. ***To cure cholera***—Boil 6 gm mint leaves and 3 gm *Ilaichi* (*Elettaria cardamomum*) in water. When water reduces to half, then cool and filter Take the water (filtrate) at an interval of 1 or 2 hours. It stops vomiting and gives relief.
2. ***To remove pimples and frackles on the face***— Grind the leaves in wine to make a fine paste. Apply it over the face.
3. ***To kill worms in nose***—Grind leaves in water and then strain. Place 2 or 3 drops in the nostrils. The worms will be killed.
4. ***To check conception in a woman***—Make a powder of dry leaves. Take 10 gm powder with water before cohabitation.

5. ***To cure migraine***—Boil two spoonfuls of dry leaves. When water reduces to half, remove heat. Add one spoonful of sugar, then strain. Drink one cup when headache occurs.
6. ***To cure dyspepsia***—It is a good home remedy for dyspepsia and indigestion when taken with black salt in form of *chatni*.
7. ***To check gas formation***—It checks gas formation, rather gives prompt relief when its *chatni* is made with unripe Amla and black salt, taken with meals daily.

5

VEGETABLES

1. Amaranth (Chaulai)

Botanical name : *Amaranthus blitum* L. Var. *Oleracea Hook. f.*

Family : Amaranthaceae

Sanskrit name : Bashpaka

Plant part used : Whole plant and leaves

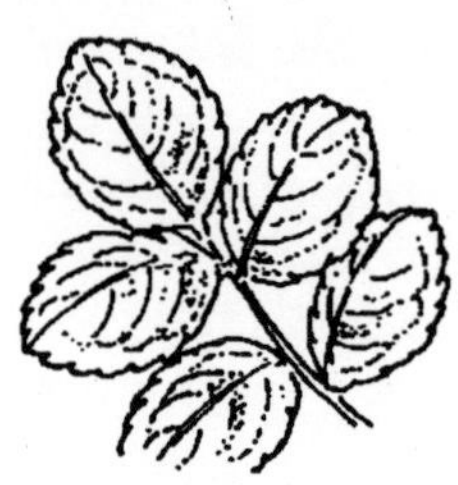

Identification

A tall, erect herb. Leaves ovate-oblong. Flowers yellowish-green, in axillary clusters. Seeds lenticular, polished.

Distribution

It is a native of Asia. It is cultivated in India, Sri Lanka, Burma, western China and Indonesia. In India, it is grown in Punjab, U.P., Himachal Pradesh, M.P. and W. Bengal.

Chemical Composition

The plant contains 85.8% moisture, 4.9% protein, 0.5% fat, 5.7% carbohydrates, 3.1% mineral matter, 0.5% calcium, 0.1% phosphorus, 21.4 mg iron, vitamins A, B_1 and C.

Medicinal Uses

1. ***To remove cataract***—Drink a cup of juice of crushed leaves daily. The cataract in the eyes will disappear.

2. ***To cure night blindness***—Cook the fresh leaves as vegetable without salt and chillies. Add *ghee* to it. Take it after the meal just after a gap of one hour.

3. ***To check excessive menstruation***—Crush fresh leaves and place in 3 cups of water. Simmer on a very low heat. Place for cooling and then strain. Drink one cup daily.

4. ***Bleeding trouble***—It is useful in all kinds of bleeding trouble. A cup of leaf juice mixed with a teaspoonful of lime juice should be taken every night in conditions like bleeding from the gums, rose, lungs, piles & also in excessive menstruation.

5. ***Leucorrhoea***—It is also useful in the treatment of leucorrhea. The root is boiled in 250 ml water and when water is reduced to 125 ml, it is decanted and taken daily morning and evening for 2/3 days as per need.

6. ***Anaemia***—It is a rich source of iron. Its vegetable should be prepared in an iron pot in order to double the iron content and be taken with each meal for a weak.

7. ***To dissolve stone***—Take the juice of fresh plants twice a day for stone trouble in urinary bladder or kidney.

8. ***To relieve swelling***—Make a paste of the amaranth plants. Apply the paste over swelling and tie with a cloth.

2. Bitter Gourd (Karela)

Botanical name : *Momordica charantia* L.

Family : Cucurbitaceae

Sanskrit name : Sushavi, Karavella

Plant part used : Fruit

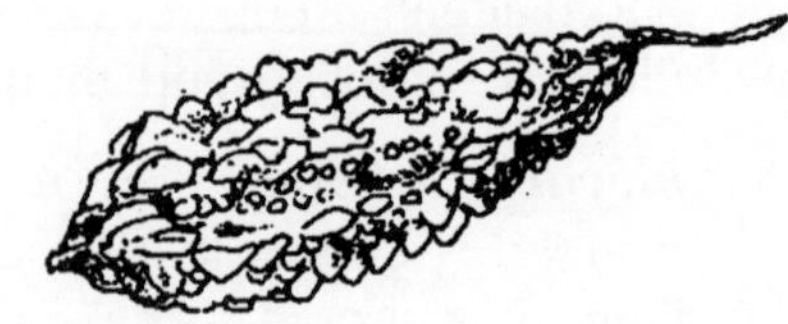

Identification

A slender creeping or climbing herb. Leaves deeply robed, reniform or sub-orbicular; flowers solitary, yellow. Fruits oblong, bitter, deeply tubercled.

Distribution

It is a native of Asia. It is now cultivated in India, Indonesia, China, Malaysia, Singapore and Burma. In India, it is grown throughout and also occurs wild.

Chemical Composition

Green fruits contain 90% moisture, 2.1% carbohydrates, 0.2% proteins, 0.3% fats, 0.9% minerals, 2.3% fibres and vitamins A, B_1, B_2 and C. Highly aromatic essential oil contains carotene, saponine, momordicine and charantin. They also contain 0.27% calcium, 0.38% magnesium and 0.64% phosphorus.

Medicinal Uses

1. ***To cure diabetes***—Crush 2 fruits to squeeze the juice. Take one cup of juice daily after breakfast. After 2 months the sugar level will be normal.
2. ***To keep sore throat fit***—Grind two dry fruits in vinegar to prepare a paste. Besmear it over the sore throat once in a day.
3. ***To cure liver and kidney ailments***—Crush fruits to squeeze juice. Take one cup juice daily. All types of

disorders related to liver and kidney will be cured within two months.

4. ***To cure dropsy***—Prepare juice from the fruits. Mix honey and juice in equal amounts. Take twice a day.
5. ***To make enlarged spleen normal***—Grind two fruits to prepare juice. Take one cup juice daily in the morning.
6. ***To cure deafness***—Cut two fruits lengthwise in small pieces. Put them in mustard oil and boil. When fruits turn ash, remove them. Store the oil in a bottle. Apply 2 or 3 drops in ears. It will improve hearing.
7. ***To remove uric acid***—It is boon for arthritis and joints pain, as it washes out uric acid easily from the body.
8. ***Gastric trouble***—For stomach disorders, its juice is effective, as it corrects the acidity, gastritis. A cup of fresh juice 3/4 times daily is helpful.

3. Bottle Gourd (Lauki)

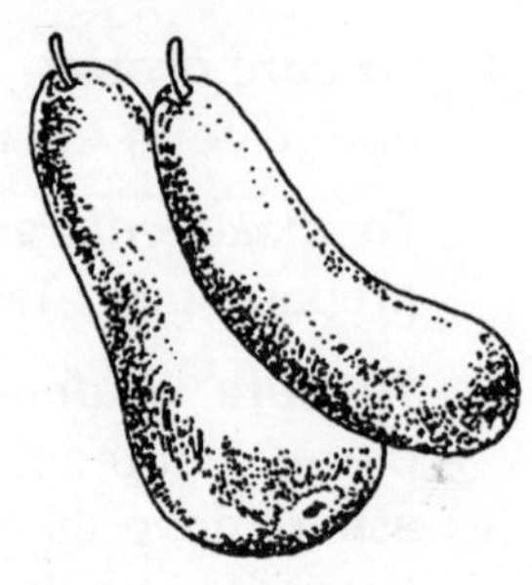

Botanical name : *Lagenaria siceraria* (Molina) Standl.
Family : Cucurbitaceae
Sanskrit name : Alabu
Plant part used : Fruit

Identification

A climbing herb. Leaves 3-5 lobed or angled. Flowers white. Fruits greenish-yellow, usually bottle or dumb-bell shaped.

Distribution

A native of Africa. One of the most ancient cultivated crops. Grown in Peru, Mexico, Egypt, India, China and New Zealand. Cultivated throughout India.

Chemical Composition

The fruit contains 96% moisture, 2.5% carbohydrate, 0.2% proteins, 0.1% fats, 0.5% minerals and 0.6% fibres. It is rich in potassium, calcium and vitamin B_1 and C.

Medicinal Uses

1. ***To cure earache***—Take stalk of fruit. Crush it and squeeze juice. Apply 2 to 3 drops in ear to stop pain immediately.
2. ***To relieve eye pain***—Cut fruit pulp in thin slices. Place one after another over closed eyelids to relieve pain.
3. ***To stop bleeding***—Remove peels and dry. Prepare powder, mix sugar candy in equal amounts and take 5 gm twice a day with water.
4. ***To cure leucorrhoea***—Cut fruit into small pieces. Take 5 pieces with cow's milk twice a day for 3 days.
5. ***To relieve heart trouble***—Squeeze the juice of fruit. Take half a cup twice a day.

4. Brinjal [Egg Plant (Baingan)]

Botanical name : *Solanum melongina* L.
Family : Solanaceae
Sanskrit name : Bhantaki
Plant part used : Fruit

Identification

It is a much-branched, spiny, perennial, erect, prickly under-shrub. Leaves ovate, lobed. Flowers violet or bluish, in extra-axillary cymes. Fruits round or elongate, purple, pendent berry.

Distribution

It is a native of India and is grown in the tropical, sub-tropical and warm regions of the world. It is the most common vegetable crop of southern Europe, southern U.S.A., Japan, Turkey, Italy, Egypt, India and Indonesia. In India, it is cultivated throughout the country.

Chemical Composition

The fruit contains 93% moisture, 4% carbohydrates, 1.5% proteins, 0.3% fats, 0.2% minerals and 1.2% fibres. It is rich in calcium, phosphorous, iron and vitamin B.

Medicinal Uses

1. ***To kill worms present in ears***—Take a dry fruit and burn it to make smoke. Apply the smoke in the ear. The worms will be expelled from the ear soon.
2. ***To lower serum cholesterol***—Cook fruits as vegetable and take it regularly in the meal. The seeds contain substance, which bind up cholesterol and take it out of the intestine. Thus, absorption of cholesterol does not occur in the blood.
3. ***To cure dropsy***—Take a fruit and make a cavity in it. Place sal-ammoniac in the cavity. Keep it in the open place for a night. Squeeze juice from it in the morning. Place 2 or

3 drops of juice in *batasha* and swallow it. The dropsy will be cured in one month.

4. ***To act as sweat preventive***—Crush the fruit and squeeze juice. Apply juice on the palm and sole. It will check perspiration. Continue it for a week.

5. ***A anti-hemorrhoidal***—It is very effective when used externally in a fat or oil-based preparation to relieve hemorrhoidal discomfort.

6. ***To relieve the hurt pain***—Crush the fruit and squeeze the juice. Mix sugar candy in the juice and take two times a day.

7. ***To cure bone-fracture***—Cut the fruit lengthwise into 2 pieces. Place salt and *haldi* (turmeric) powder on the innerside of the piece. Warm this piece and then tie on the fractured bone.

5. Broad Bean (Bakla)

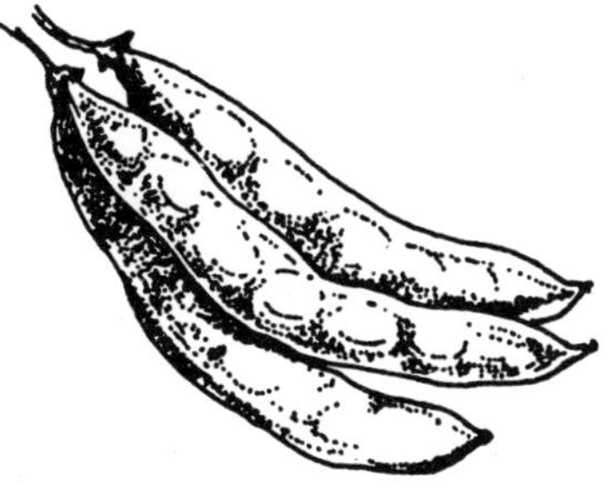

Botanical name : *Vicia faba* L.

Family : Fabacea
Papilionaceae

Sanskrit name : Bakla

Plant part used : Fruits

Identification

An erect annual herb. Leaflets 1-3 pairs, oval to oblong. Flowers dull white, with purplish spot.

Distribution

Broad bean is a native of Mediterranean region or south-western Asia. It is cultivated in Europe, China, India, Sudan, Algeria, Burma and the U.S.A. In India, it is grown throughout the country.

Chemical Composition

Fresh fruits contain 60.6% moisture, 20.4% protein, 1.5% fat, 28.4% carbohydrates, 7.1% fibre, 3.2% minerals and vitamins A, B_1 and C. Fruits also contain convicine and vicine-glucosides.

Medicinal Uses

1. ***To act as cancer preventive***—Cook broad beans as vegetable and take regularly in diet. Beans contain certain substances, which block activity of cancer-producing enzymes and prevent the growth of tumour cells.
2. ***To help diabetic patient***—Cook broad beans and take as vegetable in diet regularly. It helps maintain the blood sugar level.

6. Cabbage (Patta Gobhi, Karamkalla)

Botanical name : *Brassica oleracea* L. Var. *capitata* L.

Family : Brassicaceae cruciferae

Sanskrit name : Bandhagobhi

Plant part used : Fleshy overlapping leaves.

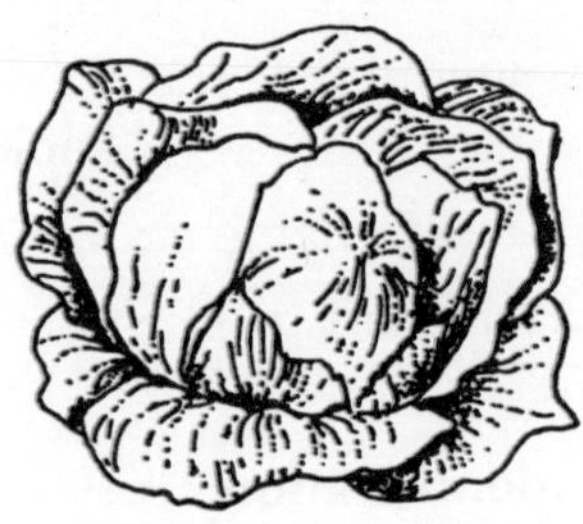

Identification

It is biennial but grown as an annual vegetable. Stem is short and stout. Leaves thick, fleshy and overlap, forming a compact round "head".

Distribution

It is believed to have originated in the cultivated Mediterranean region and southern England. It is now throughout the world, mainly in Europe, Japan, China, India, United States, Korea and Turkey. In India, it is grown as a winter crop in the plains of northern India.

Chemical Composition

Cabbage consists of 92% moisture, 4.7% carbohydrates, 1.9% proteins, 0.09% fats, 0.6% minerals. It also contains calcium, phosphorus, sodium, potassium and 1% crude fibres. Vitamins A, B_1, B_2 and C are also present.

Medicinal Uses

1. ***To act as cancer preventive***—Cook leaves as vegetable and take in diet regularly. The sulphur and histidine present in the leaves inhibit the growth of tumours and keep body cells normal.
2. ***To cure goitre***—Cut young leaves into pieces and consume them as salad regularly. It helps cure the iodine deficiency diseases.

3. ***To minimise chances of heart diseases***—Cook leaves as vegetable and take regularly in diet. The cholesterol level in blood will not increased. Therefore, the walls of the arteries will not become hard.

4. ***To give relief in gout***—Prepare a paste of leaves. Place it over the site of swelling and bind with some adhesive paste.

5. ***To check ageing***—Cabbage contains several elements & factors, which increase the immunity of the human body and prevent ageing. It also contains vitamin B and C, which give strength to the blood vessels and keep infections at bay.

6. ***To ease constipation***—Cabbage clears constipation as it is full of roughage, *i.e.* indigestible material, which is necessary to activate intestine for proper action of bowels. A meal of raw cabbage is a remedy for obstinate constipation.

7. ***To fight Alzheimer's***—Cabbage provides silicon, which interferes with the absorption of aluminium.

7. Cluster Bean (Guar)

Botanical name : *Cyamopsis tetragonoloba* (L.) Taub.

Family : Fabaceae papilionaceae

Sanskrit name : Bakuchi

Plant part used : Fruit

Identification

An erect, robust annual herb. Leaflets 3, ovate-elliptic. Flowers pinkish-purple, in axillary racemes. Fruits in erect clusters, compressed.

Distribution

It is a native of India, from where it spread to drier tropical regions of the world. It is grown in India, Pakistan and the U.S.A. In India, it is cultivated in Gujarat, Punjab, U.P., Rajasthan, M.P. and Bihar.

Chemical Composition

Pods contain 82.5% moisture, 3.7% protein, 0.2% fats, 2.3% crude fibre, 9.9% carbohydrates, 1.4% mineral matter, 0.13% calcium, 0.05% phosphorus and 5.8 mg/100 gm Iron. They also contain vitamins A and C.

Medicinal Uses

1. ***To maintain blood sugar level***—Cook fruits as vegetable and take it regularly in diet. One should have no chances of developing diabetes later in life.
2. ***To reduce obesity***—Cook fruits and take as vegetable regularly. The chemicals present in the fruit dissolve fat in the body. This helps in weight loss.

8. Lady's Finger (Bhindi)

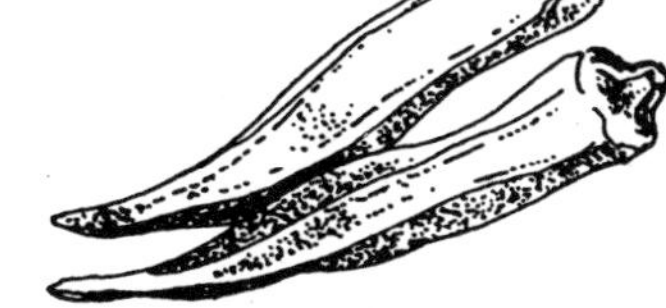

Botanical name : *Abelmoschus esculentus* (L.) *Moench.*
Family : Malvaceae
Sanskrit name : Gandhamula
Plant part used : Fruit

Identification

An erect hairy herb. Stems are green or sometimes tinged red. Leaves 3-7 lobed. Flowers large, yellow with crimson centre. Fruits is a pyramidal oblong capsule.

Distribution

It is a native of tropical Africa. It is now cultivated throughout the tropical countries of the world. In India, it is grown in U.P., Punjab, M.P., Orissa, West Bengal and Bihar.

Chemical Composition

Fruits contain 89.6% moisture, 6.4% carbohydrates, 1.9% proteins, 0.2% fats, 0.7% minerals, 1.2% fibres. They are rich in calcium, phosphorus, potassium and iodine. They also contain vitamins A, B_1, B_2 and C.

Medicinal Uses

1. ***To cure psoriasis***—Cut fruits lengthwise into pieces. Grind them to make a paste. Apply it on the skin with hand and leave for 2-3 hours. Continue with it for 15 days.
2. ***To heal burns***—Cut fruits and make a paste. The paste should be thick and slimy. Apply it over the burned part with hand. Cover it with thin cloth. After 3 or 4 hours the dressing should be changed. It will reduce the pain and swelling. Repeat it till new cells are formed.
3. ***To keep diabetic patients fit***—Cut 3 to 5 fruits lengthwise, each in 2 pieces. Keep them over night in water. Take water after removing pieces in the morning. The sugar level will be normal in one month.

9. Loofah (Torai)

A. Ghia Torai (Smooth loofah)

Botanical name : *Luffa cylindrica* (L.) M. Roem

Family : Cucurbitaceae

Sanskrit name : Rajkoshataki

Plant part used : Fruit

B. Nashili (Jinga) Torai (Angled loofah)

Botanical name : *Luffa acutangula (*L.) Roxb.

Family : Cucurbitaceae

Sanskrit name : Koshataki

Plant part used : Fruit

Identification

A climbing herb. Stem glabrous. Leaves 5-7 angled. Tendrils trifid. Flowers yellow. Fruits cylindrical (smooth loofah) or angular, 10-angled (angled loofah). Seeds ovate, compressed.

Distribution

It is a native of India. It is now cultivated all over the tropical regions of the world. It is grown in India, Malaysia, Brazil, Mexico, China and Philippines. In India, it is grown throughout the country.

Chemical Composition

An average fruit contains 93% water, 1.2% protein, 0.2% fat, 3.1% carbohydrate, 2.0% fibre, 0.5% ash and 1.0% minerals. The fruit also contains vitamins. A bitter substance luffin is present.

Medicinal Uses

1. ***To treat jaundice***—Crush fruit to squeeze juice. Mix sugar in juice and then take it two times a day.

2. ***To stop bleeding***—Grind fruit of smooth loofah to a paste. Apply it over the cut. It will stop bleeding immediately.
3. ***To cure asthma***—Crush fruit of angled loofah and squeeze juice. Mix sugar in juice and then take two times a day.
4. ***To kill worms in intestine***—Boil the fruits of angled loofah and then mix salt. Take it two times a day.
5. ***To stop dysentery***—Leaves are good substitute for ipecacuanaha in dysentery. To make it more effective, its leaves and Euphorbia hirta (Lal Duddhi) leaves are crushed together in the ratio (1:1) and taken one teaspoonful thrice a day.
6. ***To get full nutrition***—Torai contains full nutrition as a number of amino acid, vitamins and minerals are there in this fruit.

Warning

1. Do not take smooth loofah when you are suffering from dysentery.
2. Do not take angled loofah when you are suffering from phlegm.

10. Potato (Aloo)

Botanical name : *Solanum tuberosum* L.
Family : Solanaceae
Sanskrit name : Aluk
Plant part used : Underground stem, tuber

Identification

A perennial herb with underground stem, tuber. Underground steams have scale-like leaves. In the axils of these scale-like leaves, there are axillary buds, which are called the "eye" of the potato. Flowers white to blue in forking clusters. Fruits globose.

Distribution

Potato is a gift of new world. It originated in the Andes in South America. It was introduced in Europe in the 16th century. It is widely cultivated throughout the world. India is a major potato producing country. It is mainly cultivated in U.P., West Bengal and Bihar.

Chemical Composition

A tuber consists of about 80% water and 20% solid matter. Of the latter, starch is about 85% and the rest is mostly protein. Potatoes are excellent source of vitamin C. They also contain calcium, iron, magnesium, phosphorus and potassium.

Medicinal Uses

1. ***To give relief in burns***—Grind tubers into a fine paste. Besmear it over the site of burns as a plaster. It gives relief immediately.
2. ***To remove conjunctivitis***—Rub the tuber over the stone. A fine paste is left. Apply it in the eyes in the morning and evening. After 15 days, conjunctivitis will be removed.
3. ***To remove wrinkles of the face***—Grind and make a paste out of the tuber. Add paste in boiled water, so that it becomes thick. Apply thick paste over the face.

4. ***To prevent stone formation***—Cook potato tubers with rind as vegetable. Take it regularly with diet. No stones in any part of the body will be formed.
5. ***To reduce obesity***—Bake the tubers in open fire. Remove their rinds. After mixing common salt, take regularly. It will reduce fat in the body.
6. ***To cure acidity***—Crush tubers and squeeze juice. Drink one cup juice two times a day. The acidity as well as burning sensation in stomach will get cured in 15 days. Apart from it, boiled potatoes without salt is quite helpful in combating acidity.

Warning

Take potato daily in small quantity. If consumed in large quantity at a time, it may cause indigestion and intestinal disorders.

11. Pumpkin, Red Gourd (Kaddoo, Kashiphal)

Botanical name : *Cucurbita maxima* Duch. ex Lam

Family : Cucurbitaceae

Sanskrit name : Kashiphal

Plant part used : Fruit

Identification

Annual prostrate herb. Leaves circular to reniform with 5-round shallow lobes. Flowers yellow. Fruits large.

Distribution

A native of Asia. Now cultivated in India, China, Japan, Indonesia, Brazil, USA, Peru and Europe.

Chemical Composition

Fruit consists of 92.6% moisture, 1.4% protein, 0.1% fat, 5.3% carbohydrates, 0.6% mineral matter, 0.01% calcium, 0.03% phosphorus, 0.7 mg/100 gm iron and vitamins A, B_1 and C.

Medicinal Uses

1. ***To expel stone***—Select ripe fruit & squeeze juice. Add salt and take one cup juice twice a day. Repeat for 15 days. The stone in kidney or in urinary bladder will get broken and its dissolved pieces will come out through urine.
2. ***To cure migraine***—Cut fruit pulp in small pieces. Place a piece on forehead as cooling application to reduce headache. Repeat one after another till pain vanishes.
3. ***To act as cancer preventive***—Cook fruit as vegetable and consume regularly. Lowers risk of cancer.
4. ***To cure inflammation of foot sole***—Cut pulp of fruit and squeeze juice. Rubbing it over the sole gives cooling effect on the burning sensation.

12. Round Gourd (Tinda)

Botanical name : *Citrullus vulgaris* Schrad. Var. *fistulosus* (stocks) Duthie & Fuller.

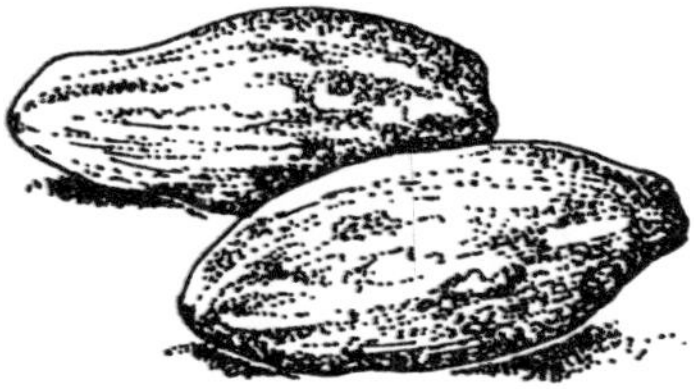

Family : Cucurbitaceae

Sanskrit name : Tinda

Plant part used : Fruit

Identification

A climbing or trailing herb. Leaves lobed. Stems and petioles fistular. Flowers yellow. Fruits light apple-green, round.

Distribution

It is a native of India. Now it is cultivated in India, Sri Lanka, Indonesia, Mexico, Africa and China. In India, it is grown in U.P., Punjab, Rajasthan and Bihar.

Chemical Composition

The fruits contain 92.3% moisture, 1.7% protein, 0.1% fat 0.6% mineral matter, 5.3% carbohydrates, 0.02% calcium, 0.03% phosphorus and 0.9 mg/100 gm iron. It also contains vitamins A, B_1 and C.

Medicinal Uses

1. ***To remove stone***—Cook fruits as vegetable and take regularly in diet. The stones present in kidney, urinary bladder and gall bladder will get broken. The small pieces of stone in later stage pass through urine.

13. Spinach (Palak)

Botanical name : *Spinacia oleracea* L.

Family : Chenopodiaceae

Sanskrit name : Palankya

Plant part used : Leaves

Identification

A vigorous, dioecious, erect biennial herb. Leaves radical, large and cauline small. Flowers unisexual.

Distribution

It is a native of South-west Asia. It was introduced in North Africa by Arabs. Now it is widely cultivated in North America, Europe and Asia. In India, it is grown in the hills and in northern states.

Chemical Composition

Spinach leaves contain 92% moisture, 3% carbohydrates, 2% proteins, 0.7% fats, 0.6% fibres and 1.7% minerals contents. It is a rich source of magnesium, sodium, potassium, sulphur and phosphorus. It also contains vitamins A and C, iodine and lecithin. It is a richer source of proteins than any other leafy vegetable.

Medicinal Uses

1. ***To protect against cancer***—Cook leaves to make vegetable. Take vegetable regularly in the meal. It inhibits tumour growth and keeps body cells normal from undergoing mutation.
2. ***To cure diabetes***—Grind leaves and squeeze juice. Take half a cup at least five minutes before each meal twice a day.

3. ***To protect eyes***—Spinach is rich in vitamin A, thus useful in promoting growth and health, especially that of eyes.
4. ***To prevent anaemia***—It is rich in iron, and thus, prevents anaemia.
5. ***To check tumour***—It is a rich source of anti-oxidant and anti-cancer compounds. It contains about 4 times more beta-carotene and 3 times more lutein than broccoli.

14. Sweet Potato (Shakarkand)

Botanical name : *Ipomoea batatas* (L.) Lamk.

Family : Convolvulaceae

Sanskrit name : Shakarkand

Plant part used : Tuberous roots

Identification

Trailing vine. Roots tuberous. Stems thin and pubecent, leaves ovate, cordate or lobed. Flowers purple, on long peduncles.

Distribution

Sweet potato is a hexaploid, unknown in wild state. It is a native of Central America and was introduced in Europe in 1492, and in China, Japan, India and Indonesia in 1698. In India, both red and white colour varieties are cultivated throughout the country.

Chemical Composition

Sweet potato contains 70% moisture, 27% carbohydrates, 0.2% fats, 1.8% proteins and 1.0% crude fibres. It also contains Vitamin A.

Medicinal Uses

1. ***To remove foreign object from the body***—Take boiled sweet potato. Its contents will get deposited around the foreign object (safety pins, coins, needles etc.), which was swallowed, accidentally. Later, it will come out with foreign object safely from the body through faces.
2. ***To protect against air pollutants***—Take roasted sweet potato regularly. Its phytochelatins can bind heavy metals in our body tissue. Thus, sweet potato protects our body against heavy metals, which we inhale from the air each day.

15. Turnip (Shalgam)

Botanical name : *Brassica rapa* L.
Family : Brassicaceae cruciferae
Sanskrit name : Shalgam
Plant part used : Roots

Identification

Herbaceous rough hairy-leaved, biennial with an enlarged root with purplish white shade. The swollen turnip root consists of hypocotyl.

Distribution

A native of central and southern Europe, it has now spread over most parts of the tropics. It was introduced in Mexico in 1586. In India, it is grown in northern parts of the country.

Chemical Composition

On an average, roots contain 91.6% moisture, 6.2% carbohydrates, 0.5% protein, 0.5% fats, 0.3% minerals and 0.9% fibres. They also contain vitamins A, B_1 and C, and 0.03% calcium, 0.04% phosphorus and 0.4 mg/100 gm iron are also present.

Medicinal Uses

1. ***To reduce cholesterol level***—Cook roots as vegetable. Take it in diet once a week. It will lower the cholesterol level in the body.
2. ***To kill worms in intestine***—Consume roots as vegetable. The worms present in intestine will get killed.
3. ***To keep constipation away***—Cut root into thin pieces and boil in small amount of water. Add lemon juice and salt according to taste. Take it once a day. It will keep constipation away.
4. ***To cure swellings of fingers***—Cut root into pieces and boil in water. Remove the pieces. When water becomes lukewarm, dip fingers inside for about half an hour. Do it twice a day. It is very effective in reducing the swellings.

16. White Goose Foot (Bathua)

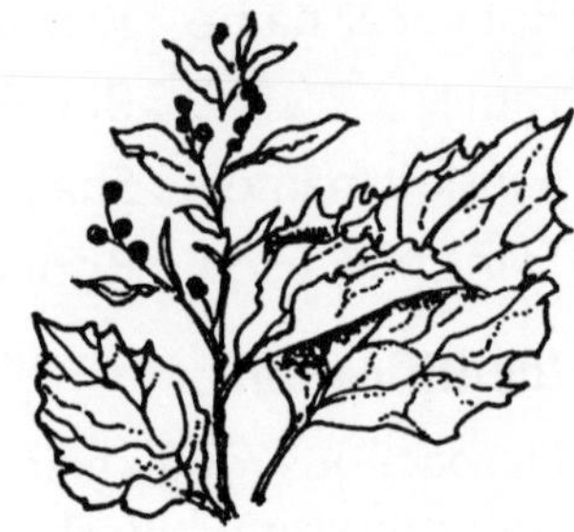

Botanical name : *Chenopodium album* L.

Family : Chenopodiaceae

Sanskrit name : Vastuk

Plant part used : Leaves and tender twigs

Identification

An erect, pubescent herb. Leaves oblong, deltoid-ovate, toothed. Flowers small, in branched spikes.

Distribution

It is a native of India. It grows as wild in the northern parts of India. It is also cultivated in the western Himalayas.

Chemical Composition

The leaves contain 81.1% moisture, 15.4% proteins, 4.05% fats, 10.6% carbohydrates, 8.1% minerals, 6.3% crude fibre, and vitamins A and C, and thiamine and riboflavin. They are also a rich source of sodium, calcium, iron and phosphorus.

Medicinal Uses

1. ***To cure gout***—Take fresh leaves and crush it to squeeze juice. Take 2 cups of juice regularly. The gout will be cured within 2 months.
2. ***To keep digestion fit***—Cook leaves and tender twigs as vegetable. Take it regularly in diet.
3. ***To kill worms in intestine***—Cook leaves as vegetable and take it. Worms of any type present in intestine will be killed.
4. ***To cure spleen and bilious disorders***—Crush young leaves and squeeze juice in small amount of water. Take one cup juice once a day. It keeps spleen and gall bladder healthy.

5. ***To act as piles preventive***—Cook leaves and tender twigs as vegetable. Take it regularly. It will check the occurrence of piles.
6. ***To expel stone out of urinary bladder***—Crush leaves in water and squeeze juice. Drink one cup juice regularly in the morning. After 15 days stone in the urinary bladder will get broken into pieces and pass through urine.
7. ***To cure leucoderma***—White spots of leucoderma can be cured or fully managed by eating *Bathua-ka-saag* and applying its juice over the spots till the season of this plant ceases.

6

OILS

1. Castor Oil (Andi, Arand)

Botanical name : *Ricinus communis* L.
Family : Euphorbiaceae
Sanskrit name : Eranda
Plant part used : Seed

Identification

An evergreen perennial shrub. Leaves palmately lobed. Flowers unisexual. Fruits regma with three seeds. Seeds have an outgrowth called caruncle.

Distribution

It is a native of India and north Africa. It is now cultivated in the tropical and sub-tropical regions of the world. The main countries are Brazil, India, Argentina, Egypt, Yemen, China and Sudan. In India, it is grown throughout the country.

Chemical Composition

Seeds contain 40-55% of non-drying oil. The oil contains 80-90% ricinoleic acid, 4.5% linoleic acid, 1.2% palmitic and stearic acids. The seeds contain toxic proteins, ricin and allergin.

Medicinal Uses

1. ***To keep digestion fit***—Add one spoonful of castor oil in warm milk. Take it at night before sleep. The constipation will go away. Repeat it whenever needed.

2. ***To regulate urination***—Add one spoonful of castor oil in warm water, take it. Regulated urination will start after half an hour.
3. ***To cure stomachache***—Mix castor oil and curd in equal amounts. Drink the mixture. Repeat it after half an hour. The pain goes away.
4. ***To treat elephantiasis***—Boil castor oil and mix *Terminalia chebula* in it. Simmer till the oil disappears. Cool and make powder. Take 3 gm powder twice a day.
5. ***To cure eye trouble***—Boil castor oil and then cool it. Soak a piece of cotton and tie it over eyelids. It will give relief in pain and inflammation.
6. ***To kill worms in intestine***—Mix the castor oil and honey in equal ratio. Take it twice a day.
7. ***To give relief in arthritis***—Rub castor oil at the site of pain twice a day. It will take one month to relieve the pain.
8. ***In amoebiasis***—Milk boiled with root powder of castor should be taken every night for regularising bowel movements and stop mucous and blood.
9. ***In gout and hernia***—The seeds of castor are crushed in milk & consumed twice a day to relieve gout pain. It is effective in hernia also.
10. The seed oil is also used for headache & cooling effect.

Warning

Crude castor oil should not be taken internally because due to ricin. It may cause harmful effects. Thus, medicated castor oil is recommended for internal uses.

2. Coconut Oil (Nariyal)

Botanical name : *Cocos nucifera* L.

Family : Palmae (Arecaceae)

Sanskrit name : Narikela

Plant part used : Copra of fruit

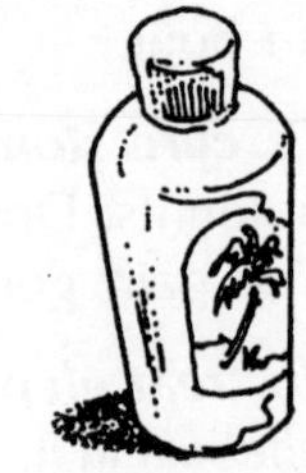

Coconut Oil

Identification

It is a tall, unbranched tree. Leaves compound. Flowers unisexual covered by spathe. Fruit ovoid, fibrous drupe. Endosperm is white, fleshy, filled with coconut milk.

Distribution

It is native of South-east Asia, from where it reached the coasts of South or Central America. The plant is now widely grown in the coastal areas of Philippines, Indonesia, Mexico, India, Papua New Guinea, Sri Lanka and Malaysia.

Chemical Composition

Copra (endosperm) consists of 60-75% oil. The oil contains many fatty acids, e.g. 48% lauric acid, 15% myristic acid, 8.5% palmitic acid, 8.0% capric acid and 6% oleic acid.

Medicinal Uses

1. ***To give relief in burn pain***—Rub coconut oil over the burnt part of the body thrice a day. It gives relief in burning sensation.
2. ***To cure eczema***—Add lemon juice and camphor powder in coconut oil. Mix them thoroughly. Rub the mixture over itching sensation two times a day.
3. ***To kill worms in intestine***—Take two spoonfuls of oil twice a day. The worms in intestine will be killed.
4. ***To cure whooping cough***—Take two spoonfuls of oil thrice a day. It will give relief immediately.

5. ***To destroy dandruff***—Mix camphor powder in coconut oil. Apply it on the head and rub with fingers at the roots of hair for 10 minutes. It will destroy dandruff and prevent baldness.

Warning

Patients suffering from asthma, bronchitis and influenza should avoid the internal use of coconut oil.

3. Linseed Oil (Alsi Ka Tel)

Botanical name : *Linum usitatissimum* Linn.
Family : Linaceae
Sanskrit name : Atasi, Nilpushpi
Plant part used : Seeds

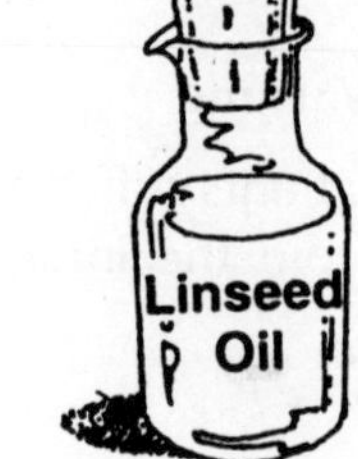

Identification

Annually cultivated herb. Leaves ovate to lanceolate. Flowers blue or white, in terminal racemes. Fruits capsule, surrounded by persistent sepals. Seeds oval, flattened, with yellow or red testa and a raphe line, black or white.

Distribution

A native of the Mediterranean and south-west Asia. Widely cultivated in India, Russia, Argentina, Pakistan, USA, China, Japan and European countries. In India, grown in M.P., Rajasthan, Karnataka, Bihar, U.P. and West Bengal.

Chemical Composition

The oil contains linolenic acid (30-60%), stearic acid and palmitic acid (6-16%), oleic acid (13-36%), linoleic (10-25%), and myristic and archidic acids. The oil also contains mucilage, proteins, wax, resin, phosphates, glycoside and lanamarin.

Medicinal Uses

1. ***To treat burns***—Mix oil with lime water in equal amounts & apply it over burns. It will give relief in pain.
2. ***To cure earache***—Place two or three drops of oil in the ear with the help of a dropper. The ache will be removed.
3. ***To melt phlegm***—Place two drops in nostril and sniff. The phlegm melts and flows out as liquid.
4. ***To use in skin diseases***—Apply linseed oil on the pimples, boils, sores etc. regularly.

4. Mustard Oil (Sarson)

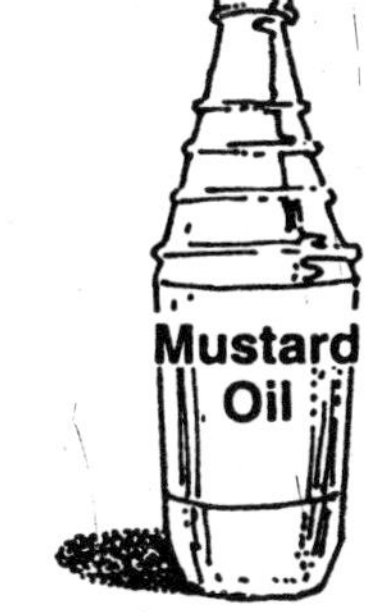

Botanical name : *Brassica campestris* L. var. *sarson* Prain
Family : Branssiaceae Cruciferae
Sanskrit name : Sarshapa
Plant part used : Seeds

Identification

A tall, erect, annual herb. Lower leaves, larger pinnatifid. Flowers yellow, in corymbs. Fruits long. Seeds yellow or brown, small and spherical.

Distribution

A native of Mediterranean region, introduced to South Asia and China. It is extensively cultivated from eastern Europe to India, China and in Africa. India is the largest producer of mustard and rape in the world. U.P., Punjab, Rajasthan, M.P. and Assam are the main mustard-producing states of India.

Chemical Composition

The seeds contain 50-67% semi-drying oil. The oil contains 45-50% erucic acid. Other important fatty acids are oleic acid, linoleic acid, palmitic acid, stearic acid and linoceric acid. A glycoside, sinigrin present in seed undergoes hydrolysis to form allyl-iso-thiocyanate, which gives pungency to the oil.

Medicinal Uses

1. ***To improve eyesight***—Rub mustard oil on the thumb of feet before taking bath every day. This will help maintain eyesight throughout the life.
2. ***To cure cough***—Mix mustard oil and *gur* (molasses) in equal amounts properly. Take it twice a day for three weeks.

3. ***To treat ringworm***—Burn a postcard to make ash and mix with mustard oil. Rub this mixture over the ringworm. It will remove the ringworm soon.

4. ***To remove burning sensation of feet***—Mix mustard oil in water and then churn. After churning, rub over the sole of feet. It will give relief in the burning sensation.

5. ***To cure hemicrania***—Put a few drops of oil in the nostril of that side of your head, which is feeling headache. Continue doing it for at least five days.

6. ***To give relief in toothache***—Mix common salt and mustard oil. Apply it over teeth and rub gently. It will subside pain and if used regularly, pyorrhoea can be cured.

7. ***To cause mosquitoes to run away***—Mix the powder of Bishop's weed in mustard oil. Dip four pieces of cardboard in this mixture and then hang them over the doors and windows. The mosquitoes will leave the room immediately.

8. ***To kill centipede***—Pour mustard oil over centipede. The animal will get detached from the human or animal body and will be killed soon.

9. ***To grow hair on bald head***—Place mustard oil in a vessel. Boil it. Add a few leaves of myrtle *(Lawsonia inermis L.)* which get burnt slowly. Now strain and store it. Rub it on the head twice a day. New hair will start growing.

10. ***To cure eczema***—Heat mustard oil and coaltar in equal amount over fire. When they boil take out and place for cooling. Rub the mixture two times a day. The eczema will be cured within a week.

5. Sesame Oil (Til)

Botanical name : *Sesamum indicum* L.

Family : Pedaliaceae

Sanskrit name : Tila

Plant part used : Seeds

Identification

An erect, hairy herb. Lower leaves deeply divided, upper leaves entire, linear-oblong. Flowers pink, solitary. Seeds black or white.

Distribution

It is a native of Africa and now cultivated in all tropical and sub-tropical countries of the world. India, Burma, Indonesia, China, Ethiopia, Sudan, Venezuela and Mexico are the main countries growing it. It is grown throughout India.

Chemical Composition

Seeds yield 45-56% semi-drying oil. The oil contains 38-50% oleic acid, 30-43% linoleic acid, 8-10% palmitic acid and 6-7% stearic acid. The oil also contains sesamin and sesamolin glycosides.

Medicinal Uses

1. ***To cure arthritis***—Place 500 gm sesame oil in a bottle, add 20 gm camphor and then fix a cork tightly. Keep the bottle in sunlight, so that camphor gets mixed in oil. Apply the mixture twice a day at the site of pain.
2. ***To heal an abscess***—Simmer 50 gm sesame oil in stewpan over fire. Add 10 gm vermilion. Stir with the ladle till the mixture appears as paste. Keep it safe. Apply it over the abscess or boil or ulcer. It will heal it within a week.
3. ***To cure chilblain***—Mix 10 gm wax in 50 gm sesame oil and then simmer over fire. Add 10 gm bitumen and heat.

When mixture becomes complete, cool it. Rub it over the heal of feet twice a day.

4. ***To remove spots of smallpox***—Boil sesame oil and then add seeds of papaya (*Carica papaya*). When seeds become ash then let it cool. Store it for use. Apply it over the face at night. The spots will be removed within one month.

5. ***To relieve a headache***—Rub sesame oil on the forehead with a piece of soft cloth. It will relieve a headache.

6. ***To remove ear disorders***—Boil water in a pan and then place a glass jar containing a small amount of sesame oil. The sesame oil becomes warm. Use it as ear drops. It will make earwax soft and easily removable.

7

CEREALS

1. Barley (Jau)

Botanical name : *Hordeum vulgare* L.

Family : Poaceae gramineae

Sanskrit name : Divya

Plant part used : Fruits

Identification

Erect, annual tufted herb. Culms 30-70 cm tall, tufted. Leaves linear-lanceolate blade, ligule membranous. Inflorescence spike of spikelets. Spikelets single flowered. Caryopsis elliptic, grooved on the inner face, cream coloured.

Distribution

It is a native of western Asia. It is extensively cultivated in temperate regions of northern hemisphere. It is grown in Russia, China, Canada, the USA, India and Mediterranean regions. In India, it is mostly grown in northern states and hilly regions.

Chemical Composition

The grain consists of 7.3% moisture, 70% carbohydrates, 12.0% proteins, 4.1% fibre and 1.8% minerals. Important amino-acids arginine, histidine, lysine, tryptophan are also present. Grains also contain magnesium, manganese, iron and copper.

Medicinal Uses

1. ***To cure arthritis***—Grow some barley grains in earthen pot. The sprouts emerge above the soil from grains. Cut

them into 2 to 3 inches. Wash and squeeze juice. The juice is delicious, energetic and helps cure arthritis.

2. ***To help in body building***—Grow some barley grains and let them develop sprouts. Cut sprouts and squeeze juice. Take one cup juice either alone or blended with other vegetable juices, like tomato or carrot, in the morning. It will help develop a good physique. Those, who take strenuous exercises for strength and muscle expansion, should take sprouts regularly as salad or drink in their breakfast.

3. ***To clean arteries and valve around the heart***—Prepare the flour with bran and take *chapatis* (Breads) regularly in meal. The grain fibres scrub away the deposits of old fat build up that have accumulated in arteries over a long period of time.

2. Maize or Corn (Makka)

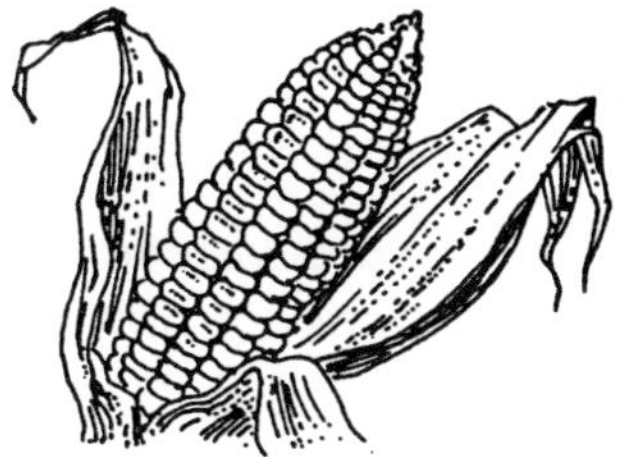

Botanical name : *Zea mays* Linn.
Family : Poaceae graminae
Sanskrit name : Yavanala
Plant part used : Fruits

Identification

An erect, herbaceous annual. Stem with distinct nodes and internodes. Leaves distichous with membranous liqule, lanceolate. Plants monoecious and diclinous. Male florets terminal, in panicles of spikelets (tassel). Female florets axillary, in spikes (cobs), enclosed by bracts. Styles long, called silk. Fruit caryopsis.

Distribution

Maize originated in South-east Asia, probably in India. It was carried to Europe by Columbus. Thereafter the Spaniards and the Portuguese introduced it throughout the tropical countries. It is extensively grown in the U.S.A., Mexico, Brazil, China, India, Argentina, France, Hungary and Italy. In India it is grown in U.P., Bihar, Punjab, Karnataka, M.P., Rajasthan and Himachal Pradesh.

Chemical Composition

On an average, grains contain 14.9% moisture, 11.1% protein, 3.6% fat, 2.7% fibres, 66.2% carbohydrate and 1.5% minerals (calcium, phosphorus, iron, magnesium, sodium, potassium, copper, sulphur and chloride). Vitamins (thiamine, riboflavin and niacin) are also present.

Medicinal Uses

1. ***To remove acne***—Mix corn flour in water to prepare a paste. Apply it on the face at night. Wash in the morning. The acne will get removed and complexion becomes more fair.

2. ***To reduce palm's smell***—Rub corn flour on both palms once in a day. The smell and oilyness of hands will go away.
3. ***To lower cholesterol level***—Consume either fresh or fried grains regularly. It will help clean the arteries and valves around the heart and cholesterol level will go down.
4. ***To cure kidney problems***—Take boiled grains every day in kidney problems.

3. Oat (Jai)

Botanical name : *Avena sativa* Linn.
Family : Poaceae graminae
Sanskrit name : Jai
Plant part used : Fruit (grain)

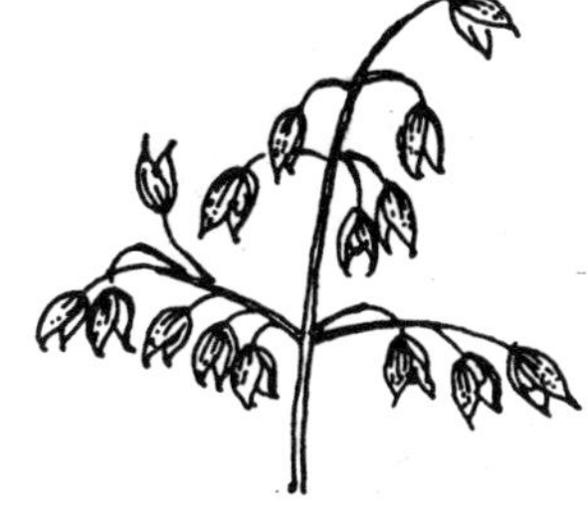

Identification

An annual tufted grass, bluish in appearance, the leaf sheath envelops the internodes, but do not have auricle at the base. Inflorescence erect or drooping. The grain is a caryopsis.

Distribution

It is a native of Asia, widely cultivated in the U.S.A., Canada, Germany, Poland, France and India. In India, it is grown in U.P., Haryana, M.P., West Bengal and Maharashtra.

Chemical Composition

The grain consists of 68% carbohydrates, 14% protein, 4.7% fats and 1% fibres. Good source of vitamin B, iron and phosphorus are also present.

Medicinal Uses

1. ***To prevent heart attack***—Boil oat grains and then filter. Take boiled grains every morning with milk in breakfast. Oat grains raise HDLs (high-density lipoproteins), which prevent heart attacks and hypertension.
2. ***To control sugar level***—Prepare chapatis of oat flour and take them in diet regularly. It will help the diabetic patients to control sugar level.
3. ***To cure psoriasis***—Boil water and add oat flour. Stir and stain. Use the water to bathe in the morning.
4. ***To use for fair complexion***—Boil one cup of water and add 6 table spoonfuls of oat flour to prepare a paste. Mix small amount of honey and the fluid of broken egg. Stir

the mixture smoothly. Apply it over the face, forehead and neck. Leave it for an hour. Wash it. The pimples, cysts, black-heads etc. will be removed. The complexion becomes fair.

4. Rice or Paddy (Chaval or Dhan)

Botanical name : *Oryza sativa* L.
Family : Poaceae gramineae
Sanskrit name : Dhanya, Shali
Plant part used : Fruit or grain

Identification

An annual herb with joined stems. Leaves alternate, linear-acuminate with a ligule. Inflorescence loose terminal panicle. Spikelets born singly with a single flower. The fruit is caryopsis, commonly called grain. Grain with husk is referred to as paddy and without husk as rice.

Distribution

It is a native of India and cultivated in Burma (Myanmar), India, Japan, China, Indonesia and Thailand. In India, it is mainly cultivated in Maharashtra, Assam, Kerala, Orissa, U.P., Bihar, M.P. and Haryana.

Chemical Composition

The grains consist of 6.1% moisture, 73% carbohydrates, 14% proteins, 4.5% fats, 1.0% crude fibres and 0.9% minerals. It is also a source of amino acids. Alkaloid oridine is present. Grains also contain traces of magnesium, manganese, zinc, iron and potassium.

Medicinal Uses

1. ***To check dysentery***—Place 50 gm rice grains in 250 gm water. Leave them to get wet for 2 hours. Now remove grains. Add sugar candy in the water. Drink two cups twice a day.

2. ***To reduce obesity***—Boil rice grains and prepare gruel. Mix common salt in gruel. Take it early in the morning. It will remove fat from the body within one month.

3. ***To stop nausea***—Place 50 gm rice grains in two cups of water. Leave them to get steep for two hours. Remove the grains and drink the water. Repeat it till nausea is stopped.

4. ***To control diarrhoea***—Boil half cup of rice grains in 3 cups of water on high heat. Filter it to remove water and leave it to cool. Take the boiled rice first and then drink the rice water. It will control diarrhoea immediately.

5. Wheat (Gehun)

Botanical name : *Triticum aestivum* L.
Family : Poaceae gramineae
Sanskrit name : Godhuma
Plant part used : Fruit

Identification

A tufted, erect annual with numerous "tillers". Leaves, have alternate arrangement. Each leaf has a basal sheath. Inflorescence spike of spikelets. Spikelets solitary 3-5 florets. Glume awned. Fruit caryopsis.

Distribution

Wheat is a native of South-west Asia. It is now cultivated throughout the world. The USA, China, India, Russia, Canada, France, Italy, Australia and Argentina are major producers of wheat. In India, it is cultivated in U.P., Punjab, Haryana, Rajasthan, Bihar, Maharashtra, Karnataka, M.P. and W. Bengal as a staple food.

Chemical Composition

Grains contain 6.9% moisture, 83% carbohydrates, 13% proteins, 3.2% fibres, 2.3% minerals and 2.1% ash. The grains also contain magnesium, manganese, zinc, iron and copper. Several amino acids are present.

Medicinal Uses

1. ***To cure hay fever***—Mix wheat bran, black pepper (*Piper nigrum*) and rock salt. Boil them in water and strain. Take filtrate at night before sleep.
2. **To keep body strong**—Boil wheat bran in two cups of water and strain. Add milk and sugar in the filtrate. Take one cup each in the morning and evening like a tea. It will help you keep away from many ailments. Bran is a relatively abundant source of dietary fibre which functions like a wet sponge in the intestine. It holds and absorbs

intoxicants and harmful compounds and carries them out of the body.

3. ***To make high blood pressure normal***—Prepare breads of wheat flour and keep them overnight, so that they become stale. Wet two stale breads in milk in the morning after breaking into pieces. They become paste like. Take them in the morning as a breakfast. It will control the blood pressure.
4. ***To treat swellings on fingers***—Mix wheat bran and common salt in water. Boil and then make it lukewarm. Place fingers of hand or foot in this water for sometime. Repeat it twice a day.
5. ***To act as a cancer preventive***—Prepare breads of wheat flour with bran and take regularly in meal. The bran inhibits the growth of tumours and prevents the chances of cancer of liver, colon and rectum. Thus, consume bran and reduce your risks of getting cancer.
6. ***To cure diabetes***—Take 7 earthen pots and fill garden soil. First day, grow some wheat grains in first pot and water it. Likewise, everyday grow some wheat grains in I-VII pots, respectively and water them regularly. The pots should be placed under protection. On next day, *i.e.* 8th day, visit 1st pot, which has well emerged sprouts above the soil. Cut and wash the sprouts and then griund them to squeeze juice. Take one cup of juice in the morning. Now remove the roots from the pot and grow some grains in it. On 2nd day, *i.e.* 9th day, visit II pot and repeat the process similar to pot I. On 3rd, 4th, 5th, 6th and 7th days repeat the same process in III, IV, V, VI and VII pots, respectively.

   Such technique may be repeated for four times and it will take one month.

   The sprouts contain growth promoting hormones, which help maintain sugar level in the body.
7. ***To heal a boil***—Prepare a thick bread of wheat flour, warm one side. On the other side, spread mustard oil (*Brassica campestris* L. var. *sarson* Prain) and then sprinkle powder

of turmeric (*Curcuma longa* L.). Place the bread in such a way that the treated side faces the boil. Tie it with a fine cloth or with adhesive tape. The redness and inflammation may disappear overnight or the boil bursts to get cured.

Warning

Consuming more wheat in diet usually causes malnutrition. The presence of a protein, glutenin, reduces the absorption of nutrients and a celiac disease develops, which causes weight loss, gas, abdominal pain and anaemia.

8

PULSES

1. Black Gram (Urad)

Botanical name : *Phaseolus mungo* Linn.
Family : Papilionaceae
Sanskrit name : Masha
Plant part used : Seeds

Identification

Annual, hairy, trailing herb with procumbent branches. Leaves trifoliate. Flowers small, yellow in clusters. Pods narrow, cylindrical, hairy with 4-10 seeds. Seeds black, rarely green.

Distribution

It is a native of India. It is now widely cultivated in India, Iran, Malaysia, East Africa and southern European countries. In India, it is grown in M.P., Punjab, West Bengal, U.P., Karnataka etc.

Chemical Composition

On an average, seeds contain 9.7% water, 23.4% proteins, 57.3% carbohydrates, 1.0% fats, 3.8% fibres and 4.8% minerals.

Medicinal Uses

1. ***To cure spermoterrhoea***—Make a powder of seeds and boil it in cow's milk. Add one spoonful of *ghee*. Take it two times a day.

2. ***To provide strength***—Add seeds in *ghee* and then fry. Boil them in cow's milk. Add sugar. Take it two times a day. It will give vital strength to body.

3. ***To treat abscesses***—Soak seeds in water and then prepare poultice. Plate it above the abscess two times a day. It will heal it in one week.

2. Gram (Chick Pea) [Chana]

Botanical name : *Cicer arietinum* L.

Family : Fabaceae

Sanskrit name : Chanaka

Plant part used : Seeds

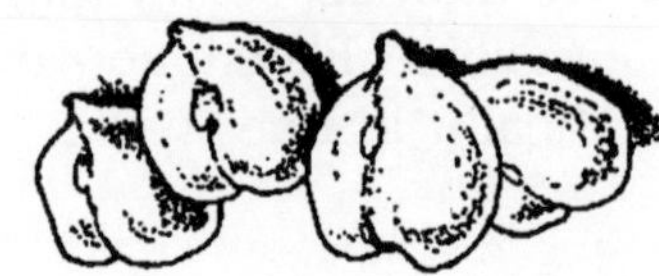

Identification

A profusely-branched hairy annual herb. Leaves imparipinnate compound. Flowers solitary axillary. Pop or legume is small and inflated or swollen.

Distribution

Originated in western Asia. Introduced to tropical America, Africa and Australia. In India, the crop is grown in U.P., Punjab, Bihar, M.P. and Haryana.

Chemical Composition

An analysis of dry seeds gives 9.8% moisture, 61.2% carbohydrates, 17.1% proteins, 5.3% fats, 3.9% fibres and 2.7% ash. The gram seeds contain oxalic, acetic and malic acids. Arginine, tyrosine, lycine, cystine and tryptophan amino acids are also present. Vitamins A, D, and E are present in the seeds.

Medicinal Uses

1. ***To relieve diabetes***—Make flour of the gram seeds and prepare *chapatis*. Take *chapatis* in meal daily for a week. It will stop the sugar in urine.

2. ***To cure sprain of heel***—Tie gram seeds at the site of twist with the help of white cloth. Pour water over gram seeds regularly. The seeds will imbibe and swell up. The sprain will be cured.

3. ***To make body strong***—Make three packages of gram seeds in white cloth. Tie one on first day, 2nd on second day and 3rd on third day above the ground. Keep them

wet regularly by pouring water. The seeds will germinate. On fourth day, visit the first package and take the seeds with their germlings early in the morning. On fifth day, take 2nd package and on sixth day take 3rd package. Repeat the process regularly for two months. It will help increase stamina and physical strength of the body.

4. ***To treat ringworm***—Grind gram seeds in water. Mix 2 spoonfuls with honey. Apply the mixture above ringworm twice a day. The ringworm will be destroyed in a week.

5. ***To destroy acne of the face***—Mix gram flour, turmeric (*Curcuma longa* L.) and curd in equal amounts to make a paste. Apply it over the face at the time of sleep and wash in the morning.
6. ***To cure intestinal disorders***—Leaves and fruit have sour taste due to the presence of oxalic and malic acids. These secretion is collected by covering the plant at night with a cloth. The acids obtained thus are used as medicine for intestinal disorders.

3. Pea (Matar)

Botanical name : *Pisum sativum* L.
Family : Fabaceae
Sanskrit name : Satila
Plant part used : Seeds

Identification

A climbing or trailing annual herb. Leaves pinnate compound with foliaceous stipules, terminating by branched tendrils. Flowers white-pinkish. Pods contain 4-10 seeds.

Distribution

A native of West Asia and Mediterranean region, it spread to Europe, India and China. Extensively cultivated in northern hemisphere: Europe, Russia, India, North-west America and China. In India, it is grown in U.P., Bihar, M.P. and Maharashtra.

Chemical Composition

Dry seeds contain 10.6% moisture, 58.5% carbohydrates, 22.7% proteins, 1.0% fats, 4.3% fibres and 3.0 minerals. Seeds also contain traces of magnesium, manganese, iron and zinc. An alkaloid, trigonelline, is also present.

Medicinal Uses

1. ***To clean arteries***—Boil green pea seeds and add common salt and red peppers. Take them regularly in refreshment. Pea seeds contain plant proteins called lectins, which have clot dissolving property. Take more green pea seeds if more susceptible to clots due to poor blood circulation.
2. ***To remove marks of chicken pox***—Boil pea seeds in water and then filter. Wash the face regularly with the boiled water. It will remove the pit marks of chicken pox and measles in children's skin.

4. Pigeon Pea (Arhar)

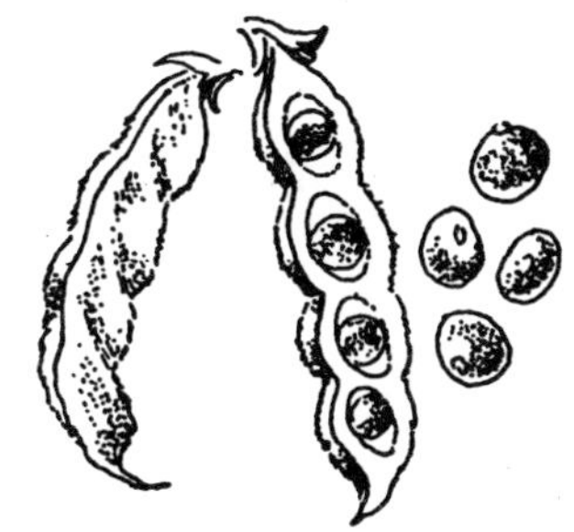

Botanical name : *Cajanus cajan* (L.) Millsp.

Family : Papilionaceae fabaceae

Sanskrit name : Adhaki

Plant part used : Seeds

Identification

A much-branched shrub. Leaves trifoliate, stipulate. Flowers yellow or purple, in terminal panicle. Fruits long. Seeds chocolate red.

Distribution

It is a native of Africa and was introduced in Syria and India through Egypt. It is now cultivated in Africa, Central America, Australia and India. In India, it is grown in U.P., Bihar, M.P., Andhra Pradesh, Tamil Nadu and Maharashtra.

Chemical Composition

Dry seeds contain 15.1% moisture, 22.3% proteins, 57.3% carbohydrates, 1.5% fat, 8.1% fibres, 3.8% ash. Seeds also contain traces of magnesium, iron, zinc and manganese.

Medicinal Uses

1. ***To cure itch***—Grind pigeon pea seeds and mix with curd to prepare a paste. Apply it over the itching sensation twice a day. It will cure the itching in four days.

9

NATURAL PRODUCTS

1. Alum (Phitkari)

Sanskrit name : Phitkari

Source : *It is prepared by concentrating solution of potassium sulphate and aluminium sulphate to cristallisation point. On cooling, alum is obtained. Potash alum is very common.*

Alum

Medicinal Uses

1. ***To stop bleeding from the nose***—Dissolve 50 gm alum in water to make a solution. With the help of cotton, drop it into the nostrils. The bleeding will stop.
2. ***To cure jaundice***—Fry a small part of alum and grind it to form a powder. Divide it into seven packages. Take one package with curd daily.
3. ***To relieve cough***—Mix alum with double amount of sugar candy. Grind them to make a powder. Divide it into 15 packages. Take one package daily with water or milk. It will give relief soon from cough.
4. ***To heal abscess***—Fry alum and then grind it as a powder. Place it inside abscess. Repeat it for 4 to 5 days.

5. ***To dispel rats***—Grind alum to make a powder. Place the powder on and around the holes. The rats will run away.
6. ***To treat internal injuries***—If any part of the body is injured internally, then take powder of 3 gm alum in one glass of milk.
7. ***To cure cholera***—Dissolve alum in fresh water to make a solution. Drink this solution thrice a day. It will give relief.
8. ***To stop oozing of sweat from palm and sole***—Dissolve alum in fresh water to prepare solution. Apply this solution on palm and sole regularly.
9. ***To act as an anti-malarial drug***—Fry alum and then grind as powder. Mix 1 gm powder and 1 gm sugar candy. Take mixture 3 hours before the time of fever. Repeat it for 5 days.
10. ***To give relief in piles***—Grind alum as powder. Mix powder with butter. Apply the mixture on glands of piles twice a day. The glands will dry and fall.
11. ***To act as antiseptic***—After shave, rub a piece of alum with water over the face.

2. Ghee (Ghee)

Sanskrit name : Ghrit

Source : *Ghee obtained from animal's milk is called Desi Ghee. Ghee made artificially with the hydrogenation of groundnut oil (Arachis hypogea L.) is called vegetable ghee.*

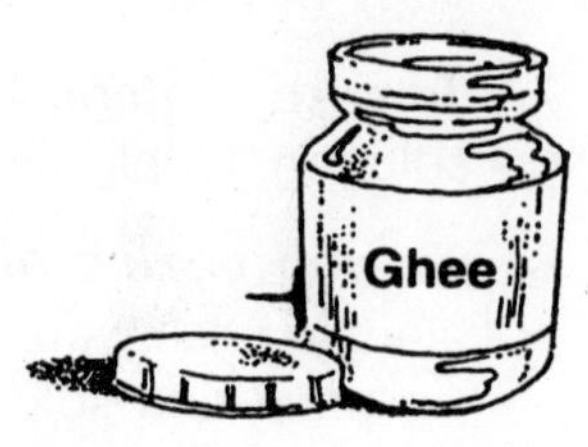

Medicinal Uses

1. ***To cure earache***—Boil *ghee* and camphor and then store in a bottle. Apply two drops in ear by a dropper. The earache will be cured.
2. ***To control urticaria***—Make a powder of mineral salt and mix it with *ghee*. Rub this mixture on the body. The urticaria will get controlled.
3. ***To take care of chilblain***—Boil *ghee* and then mix bitumen and wax. Apply this mixture to the heel of a foot. The chilblain will be cured.
4. ***To remove mouth sores***—Take *ghee* in mouth at night before sleep. Keep it in mouth. *Ghee* will not be there in mouth in the morning. Repeat it for 4 to 5 days. All the oral problems, like bad breath, sores, gum disorders etc. will be removed.

3. Honey (Madhu, Shahad)

Sanskrit name : Madhu

Source : *Bees collect nector from different flowers and store it in the holes of hive. First it is liquid and tasteless but later on becomes viscid fluid and sweet.*

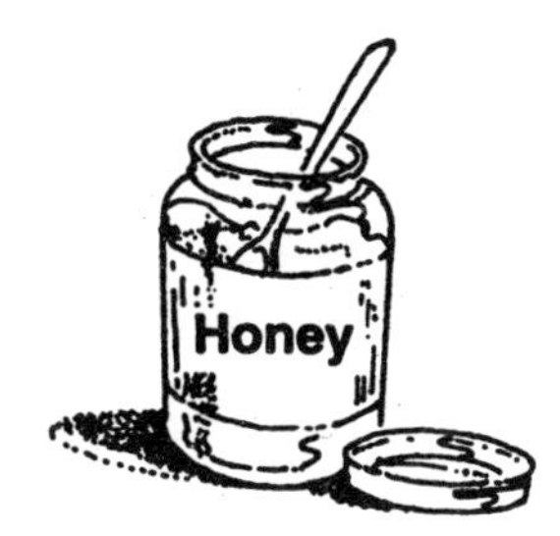

Medicinal Uses

1. ***To keep eyes fit***—Dip a basal part of glass needle in honey and then apply it to both eyes once a day. It will cure ailments and improve the eyesight.
2. ***To cure cough***—Prepare one spoonful juice of ginger and mix it with one spoonful of honey. Take it thrice a day. It will give relief by diluting the phlegm.
3. ***To remove wrinkles of the face***—Wash your face with warm water and wipe with towel. Apply a thin honey mash. Wash it again after one hour. It will give softness and fresh beauty to the face.
4. ***To heal major wounds***—Apply honey two or three times daily on the wounds. Place cotton and then tie with white clean cloth. It will check bacteria and heal wounds earlier.
5. ***To provide undisturbed sleep***—Mix one spoonful honey and one spoonful of lemon juice in half a glass of fresh water. Take it at night before sleep. It will provide a sound sleep.
6. ***To cure intestinal disorders***—Mix one spoonful of honey in one glass of fresh water. Stir and then take it two times a day. It will improve the digestion and also cure diarrhoea

and dysentery. If it is taken regularly, the obesity will be reduced.

7. ***To increase obesity***—Those who want to be more bulky should take one spoonful of honey with one glass of milk twice a day regularly. After one or two months, body-weight will increase.

8. ***To maintain normal blood pressure***—Squeeze juice from 3-4 cloves of garlic. Mix it with one spoonful of honey and take twice a day.

9. ***To treat hay fever***—Squeeze half spoonful juice from basil leaves (*Ocimum sanctum*). Mix it with one spoonful of honey and take thrice a day.

10. ***To make teething easy***—Apply honey on the gums of a baby twice a day with finger. It makes teething easy in baby.

11. ***To keep impotence away***—Squeeze juice from onion and mix it with 2 spoonfuls of honey. Take it twice a day for 21 days.

Warning

1. Do not mix honey and *ghee* in equal amounts because their mixture becomes a poison. If someone is interested in taking them, then mix in unequal amounts. Mixture of more *ghee* and less honey is safe.

2. Do not take honey alone, because it has harmful effects on the body. Thus, mix it with water or juice or any drink. Do not mix with egg, fish, meat, oil and sugar.

3. Do not take honey after warming up or with any warm foodstuff. After being warmed, the honey becomes poisonous.

4. Do not take honey in large amounts and for a long period in place of medicine, as it turns out to be a poison.

4. Kerosene Oil (Mitti Ka Tel)

Sanskrit name : Mrittika Tailam

Source : *Kerosene is obtained as a fraction when crude oil undergoes the process of refining of petroleum in a refinery.*

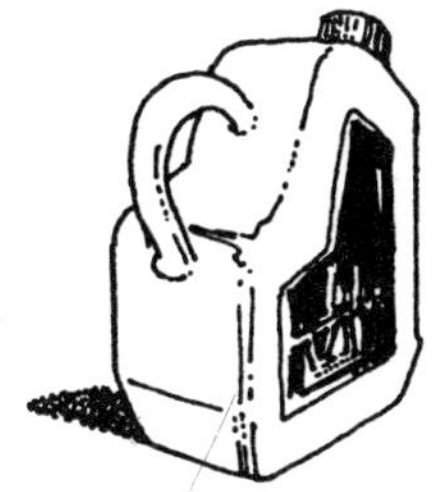

Kerosene Oil

Medicinal Uses

1. ***To stop bleeding from cuts***—Dip white cloth in kerosene and tie it over the cut. Bleeding will stop immediately. Repeat it 3 to 4 days, the cut gets healed.
2. ***To cure pyorrhoea***—Take a sip of kerosene and keep it in mouth for sometime. Then spit. Wash your mouth with water. Repeat it twice a day. Pyorrhoea and other dental disorders will be cured.
3. ***To kill lice in hair***—Apply kerosene in hair before sleep. Cover head with a cloth and leave like that for the whole night. In the morning, wash your hair. All the lice will be killed.
4. ***To give relief in wasp sting***—If a wasp has stung, then put kerosene on the sight of pain. Rub it gently. It will give relief immediately and check the swelling.
5. ***To minimise sciatica pain***—Dissolve camphor powder in kerosene. Keep this mixture in a bottle and place it under sunlight. Rub the mixture at the sight of pain slowly and then warm. The pain will be minimised.
6. ***To cure goitre***—Place a few drops of kerosene in *batasha*. Take it two times a day. Goitre will get cured.

5. Salt (Namak)

Sanskrit name : Lavan

Source : *There are 3 sources of salt: **mineral salt** (sendha namak) is obtained from the rock present in Sindh, Pakistan. **Common salt** (sadharan namak) is obtained from sea water after evaporation. **Black salt** (kala namak) is obtained from rocks.*

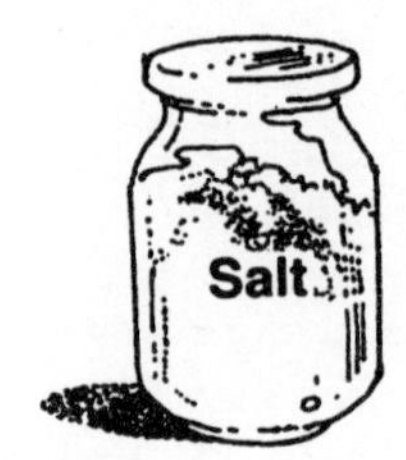

Medicinal Uses

1. ***To cure sore throat***—Boil a glass of water and add one spoonful of salt. When the mixture becomes lukewarm then do gargles 2 or 3 times a day.

2. ***To remove phlegm***—Place salt in white cloth and make a package. Warm it over the round plate of iron. Then place it over the chest at different sites. Repeat it for as many times as you like. It will help in removal of phlegm and will give relief in cough, cold and pneumonia.

3. ***To make gum strong***—Mix salt with mustard oil (*Brassica campestris* L. var. *sarson* prain) and apply the mixture over gums gently with a finger. Keep the mixture and move it slowly in the mouth. Spit after half an hour. Repeat it for 2-3 days in a week for some time.

4. ***To eliminate rheumatic pain***—In a kettle, boil Bishop's weed (*Trachyspermum ammi*), sprague and salt in water. Place a gauze above the kettle. Take a wet cloth and warm it slowly over the gauze. Apply this warm cloth above the site of pain. It will give relief in the pain. Repeat it 3 to 4 times a day.

5. ***To control cough***—Place a piece of black salt in mouth. Do not chew it. Let it dissolve slowly in mouth. It will control the cough.
6. ***To expel centipede from the ear***—If centipede has entered in any ear, then drop solution of salt with the help of dropper. The centipede will be expelled immediately.
7. ***To give relief in injuries***—Dip the injured part of body in salt solution. It subsides pain and reduces swelling.

6. Water (Pani)

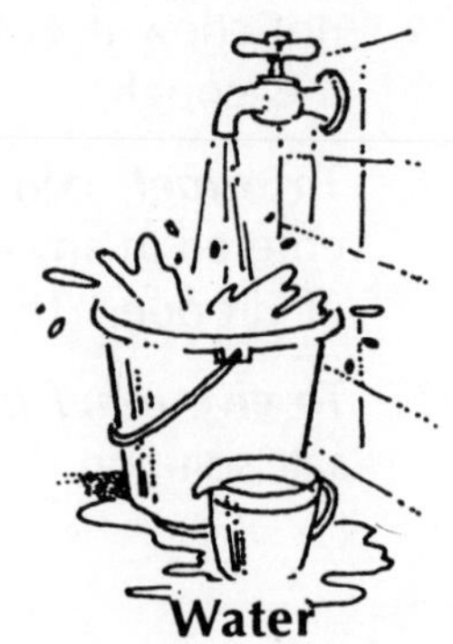

Sanskrit name : Jal

Source : *Fresh water is available in well, river and pond and also obtained from hand-pump and tubewells.*

Medicinal Uses

1. ***To eliminate constipation***—Drink 3 or 4 glasses of fresh water early in the morning before sun rise. It will help eliminate the chances of constipation and other intestinal disorders.
2. ***To cure coryza***—Boil water and then place for cooling. When warm, sip it slowly. It will give relief in cold.
3. ***To keep eyes fit***—Splash fresh water in the eyes early in the morning daily. The eyes will remain fit and eyesight will improve.
4. ***To cure anuresis***—Place boiled water in a tub and when water is warm, sit in such a manner that your waist remains dipped. Sit for half an hour twice a day. The stopped urination will restart soon.
5. ***To protect against sunstroke***—Keep your belly full of water when you are out during summer noon. You will not be affected by high temperature.
6. ***To keep cold away***—Suck the fresh water through nose early in the morning daily. One will not suffer from cold for ever.

Miracles of Water Therapy

1. I might sound incredible, but facts cannot be denied too. As said by Confucius nearly 2500 years back, the health of an organism is tempered wholly by the mechanics of the stomach. As a modern saint, Paramahansa Yoganananda, analysed that it is overeating (or eating on all the 365 days of an year) that leads to and complicates diseases.
2. Before discussing the details, one might be interested to know some of the diseases, which can be cured by this therapy.
3. Headache, hypertension, anaemia, rheumatism, general paralysis, obesity, arthritis, sinusitis, tachycardia, anesthesia.
4. Cough, asthma, bronchitis, pulmonary tuberculosis, meningitis, hepatic diseases, urogenital diseases, hyperacidity, gastritis, dysentery, rectal prolapses, constipation, hemorrhoids, diabetes.
5. Eye troubles, epthalmia haemorrhage opthalmia, irregular menstruation, leucorrhoea, uterine cancer, cancer of the mammary glads, rhinitis laryngitis etc.
6. How can one practise water therapy? Every morning as soon as one gets up, what one has to do is not wash one's mouth and face but drink 1.26 kg (1260 c.c.) of water at a stretch. Only then should one wash one's face.
7. For the next 45 minutes one should not eat nor take beverages.
8. All this should be preceded by some preparations. After the dinner, one should not eat nor drink stimulating beverages or soft drinks.
9. While following this therapy, one should drink water two hours after a meal. One should not consume any drinks containing poison or snacks/fast food before going to bed.

10. Where water contains impurities, it should be boiled in the night to be used in the morning.
11. Experience has shown that following disease were cured by water therapy within the time shown below:-

Hypertension	One month
Gastricpatosis	Two Months
Constipation	One month
Diabetes	One week
Cancer	One month
Pulmonary tuberculosis	Three months

12. Person suffering from arthritis and rheumatism should use water therapy three times a day for one week and thereafter, once a day.

Warning

Do not drink water just before meal or just after meal or even during meal. It will have harmful effects. Take water one hour after meal. It will help in the digestion of food.

10

FOOD TIPS—DO'S & DON'TS

1. Fruits are essential in diet. Take them after two hours of meal during daytime.
2. Boil water and mix a little salt and take it when it is lukewarm in place of tea. It will help dissolve oily and greasy substances.
3. Avoid drinking water during meal because it will dilute the digestive enzymes. Take it one hour after meal.
4. Go for urination just after taking meal regularly.
5. Sleep lying left side for sometime just after taking meal. It will help improve digestive system.
6. Avoid running or going on a long walk just after taking meal.
7. Drink fresh water before sunrise early in the morning when you leave the bed.
8. Soak gram (*Cicer arietinum*) seeds in water and keep them overnight. Take them in the morning regularly. Diabetic patients should consume gram seeds after getting them roasted during daytime.
9. Make it a habit to consume salad with meal. It will provide additional nutritive elements.
10. Take the fruits of *kakri* (*Cucumis melo*). It will help digest wheat. Avoid taking it empty stomach.
11. Roast wheat bran and mix two spoonfuls of sugar. Take it with warm water daily before sleep.
12. Consume less salt and sweets after the age of 40 years.
13. Take an apple daily for one month. It will remove the brain's weakness and insomnia.

14. To take vegetable of pointed gourd or *Parwal* (*Trichosanthes dioica*) is suitable in the months of rainy season. It helps control *tridoshas,* namely *vayu, pitta* and *kapha.*
15. Drink milk just after eating mango.
16. Those suffering from diarrhoea should take curd, butter, goat's milk, dry ginger and water.
17. Those suffering from bronchitis should take cow's milk, honey, mash, brinjal, garlic and ginger.
18. Avoid drinking wine, consuming tobacco and smoking when you are suffering from cancer.
19. Take cooked vegetable of unripe papaya fruit. It makes liver healthy.
20. Those suffering from indigestion should not take bitter gourd.
21. Do not take milk and fish at a time. It will cause skin diseases.
22. Do not take milk and salt or sour dishes some time.
23. Do not consume sugar, *ghee,* butter, resins, grapes, banana, groundnut, rice, potato's preparations, almond, cashew nut and *cheeku* or sapodilla (*Achras zapota*) when you are suffering from diabetes.
24. Do not consume vegetable of angled loofah (*Luffa acutangula* when you are suffering from dysentery because it creates froth in feces.
25. Do not consume the fruits of jambos (*Syzygium cumini*) in large quantity, because they cause pain in chest and create gastric trouble.
26. Do not take grapes when you are suffering from skin diseases.
27. Do not eat potato in any form during the rainy season because starch causes warmth in body.
28. Do not consume the vegetable of jack fruit (*Artocarpus heterophyllus* Lamk.) if you are suffering from dyspepsia.

29. Do not take more salt because your hair will start falling, resulting in baldness.
30. Do not take vegetable of smooth loofah (*Luffa cylindrica* when you are suffering from phlegm.
31. Do not take tea empty stomach. Take one to two cups only per day.
32. Do not take curd in the evening or at night, because it may cause cough and cold.
33. Take small cardamom (*Elettaria cardamomum*) after taking banana fruits.
34. Take meal only once during rainy season. It will keep digestion normal.
35. Before having mangoes, place them in water for 3 to 4 hours.
36. Do not consume leafy vegetables in August and September.
37. Drink more water when you have consumed rice in diet.
38. Purchase vegetables which have insect-bitten leaves. They are safe as they have not been poisoned by toxic fertilisers.
39. Mix husk of the seeds of mung (*Phaseolus aureus*) with wheat flour. Prepare *chapatis* and take them during the rainy season.
40. Do not use mustard oil in the preparation of vegetable or other dishes during March-April.
41. Do not take bitter gourd during the months of September and October.

GLOSSARY

antipruritic relieves itching.

antipyretic prevents or reduces high temperatures.

antiseptic destroys germs and microorganisms that produce disease.

antispasmodic relieves or prevents involuntary muscular spasms.

antitussive relieves coughing.

aperitif encourages the appetite.

aromatherapy a method of treatment using essential oils.

astringent a medicine that reduces the flow of secretions and discharges.

biliary deobstruent promotes the flow of bile.

bitter a bitter principle which acts on the mucous membranes of the mouth and stomach to increase appetite and promote digestion.

bradycardia abnormally slow heartbeat.

cardiotonic has a tonic effect on the heart.

carminative expels gas from the intestines.

corm big tuber.

decongestant relieves congestion.

diuretic promotes the flow of urine.

elixir a liquid preparation consisting of the extract of a potent or unpleasant-tasting medicinal plant made palatable by adding aromatic substances and honey or sugar.

emetic induces vomiting.

emmenagogue, emmanagogic restores the menstrual flow.

emollient softens the skin.

febrifuge reduces high temperatures.

galactagogue, galactagogic a medicine to increase the flow of milk in nursing mothers.

hepatoprotective protects the liver.

herbalist a person who is knowledgeable about medicinal plants.

homoeopathy therapy based on the concept of a close similarity between disease and remedy.

hypoglycaemic reduces the level of sugar in the blood.

hypotensive reduces high blood pressure.

laxative relaxes the bowels and has a gentle evacuant action.

lipid a preparation with a fatty excipient as a base, greasy to the touch and insoluble in water.

narcotic a medicament that causes drowsiness.

nephritis inflammation of the kidneys especially in Bright's Disease.

ophthalmic relative to eye diseases.

oxytocic a medicinal drug used to hasten parturition or stimulate uterine contractions.

phytotherapy therapy by means of medicinal (officinal) plants.

rhizome an underground stem which acts as a storage organ.

soporific induces sleep.

spirit solution the product obtained from alcoholic maceration of medicinal herbs. Known also as tincture.

stomachic aids the stomach action.

synergic the combined effect of certain substances that exceeds the sum of their individual effects.

tincture a spirit solution.

trachoma an infection of the eyes or throat.

urogenital pertaining to the urinary and genital organs.

BIBLIOGRAPHY

1. Anonymous (1948-52). *Wealth of India.* **Vols. I to X,** New Delhi.
2. Atal, C.K. and B.M. Kapoor (1977). *Cultivation And Utilization Of Medicinal and Aromatic Plants.* R.R.L. Jammu Tawi.
3. Chopra, R.N., S.L. Nayar and I.C. Chopra (1956). *Glossary of Indian Medicinal Plants,* C.S.I.R., New Delhi.
4. Jain, S.K. (1975). *Medicinal Plants,* New Delhi.
5. Kapoor, L.D. (1990). *Hand Book of Ayurvedic Medicinal Plants.* C.R.C., Florida.
6. Kirtikar, K.R. and B.D. Basu (1935). *Indian Medicinal Plants,* Allahabad.
7. Majumdar, A., C.P. Shukla, R.S. Josh and V.N. Pandey (1978). *Hand Book of Domestic Medicine And Common Ayurvedic Remedies.* C.C.R., New Delhi.
8. Satyavati, G.V., M.K. Raina and M. Sharma (1976). *Medicinal Plants of India.* **Vols. 1-3.,** ICMR, New Delhi.
9. Srivastava, R.C. (1989). *Drug-Plant Resources of Central India (An Inventory).* Today and Tomorrow's Printers and Publishers, New Delhi.
10. Wagner, H. (1981). *Natural Products as Medicinal Agents.* Hippocrats, Stuffgart.
11. Chief, R. 1984, Medicinal Plants, Mac Donald, London.
12. Dahanukar, S., 1995, Heal With Herbs CSIR, New Delhi.

PARENTING

FAMILY & RELATIONS

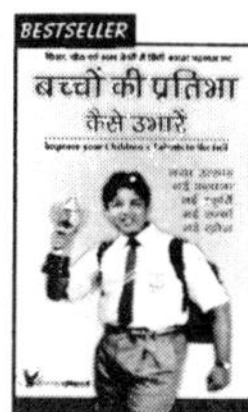

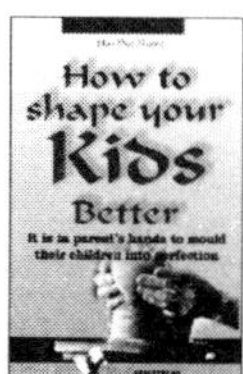

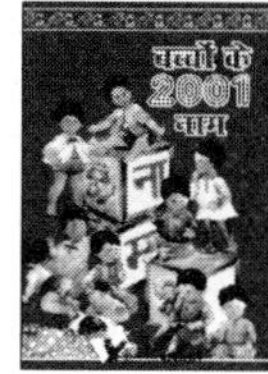

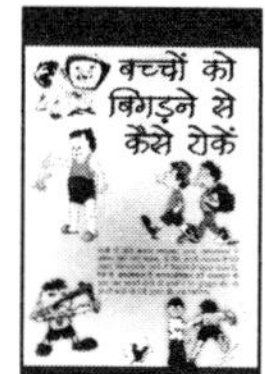

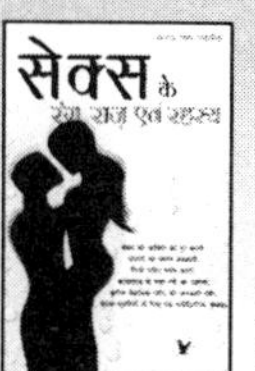

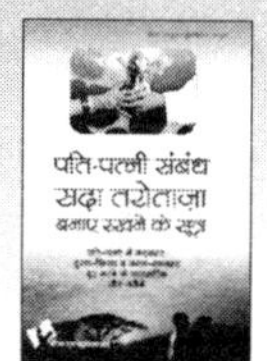

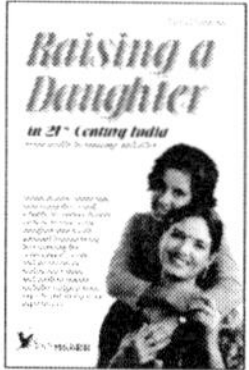

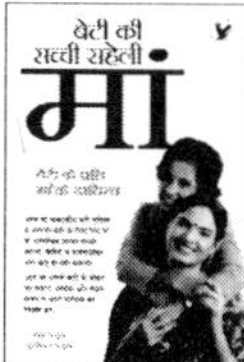

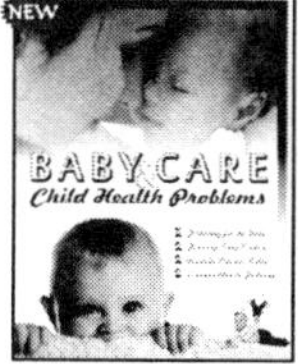

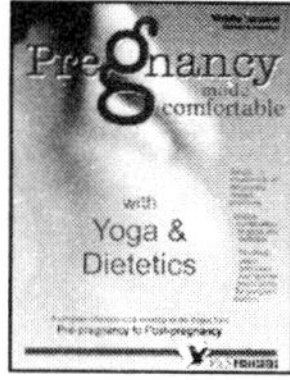

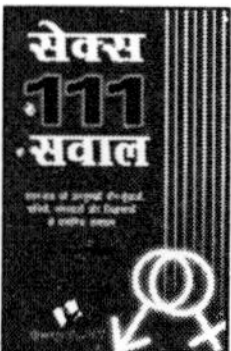

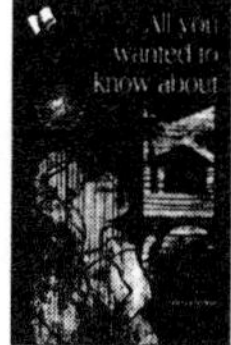

COOKING

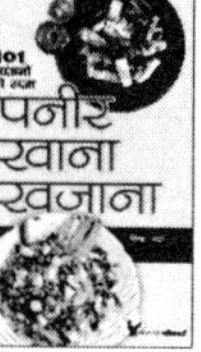

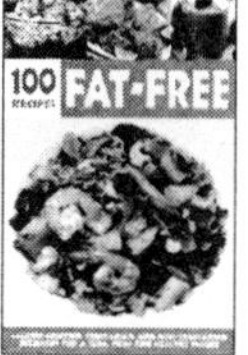

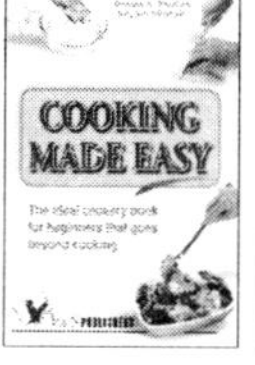

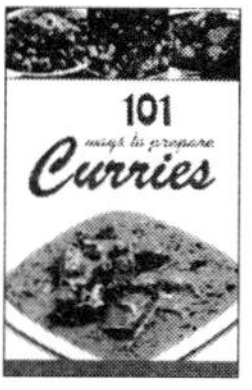

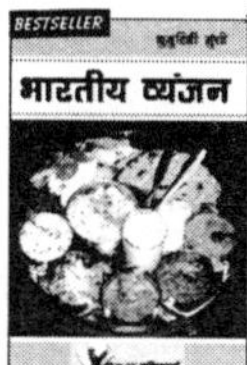

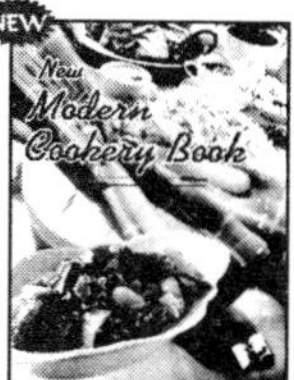

HOUSEKEEPING

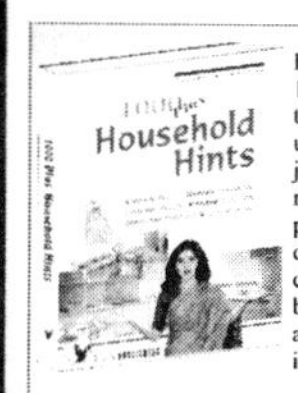

Homely guide to 1000 + domestic tips to keep skin shining, utensils clean, jewellery sparkling, rectifying small plumbing & electrical defects, keeping clothes moth-free, banish nasty smells and dressed-up interiors neatly.

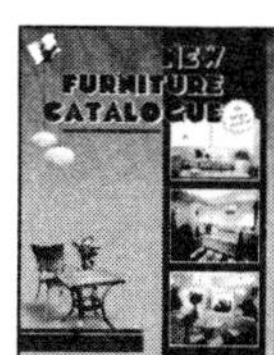

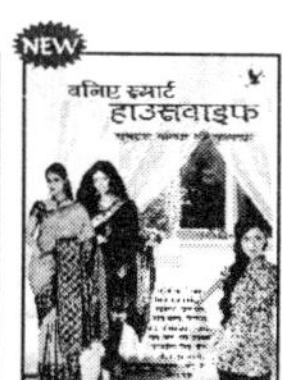

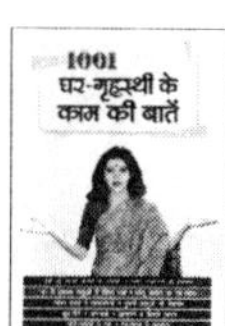

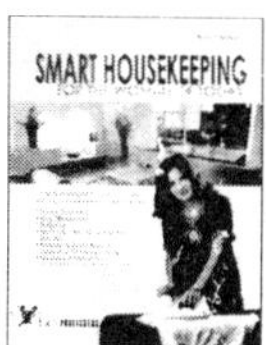

WOMEN ORIENTED

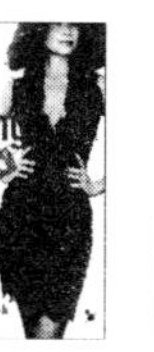

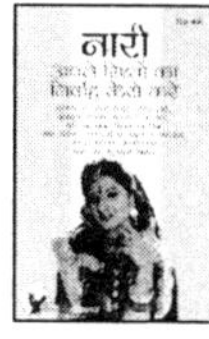

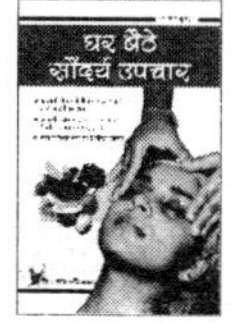

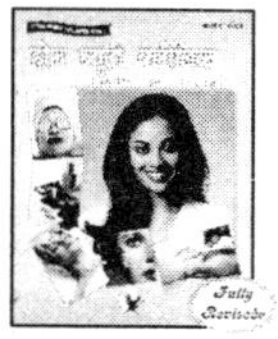

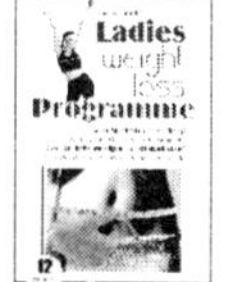

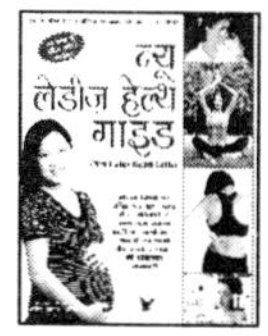